Countering the Pandemic Threat Through Global Coordination on Vaccines

The Influenza Imperative

Peter Sands and Janelle Winters, *Editors*

Committee on Global Coordination, Partnerships, and Financing Recommendations for Advancing Pandemic and Seasonal Influenza Vaccine Preparedness and Response

Board on Global Health

Health and Medicine Division

A Consensus Study Report of

The National Academies of
SCIENCES · ENGINEERING · MEDICINE
and
NATIONAL ACADEMY OF MEDICINE

THE NATIONAL ACADEMIES PRESS
Washington, DC
www.nap.edu

THE NATIONAL ACADEMIES PRESS 500 Fifth Street, NW, Washington, DC 20001

This activity was supported by a contract between the National Academy of Sciences and the Office of Global Affairs with the U.S. Department of Health and Human Services. Any opinions, findings, conclusions, or recommendations expressed in this publication do not necessarily reflect the views of any organization or agency that provided support for the project.

International Standard Book Number-13: 978-0-309-08870-1
International Standard Book Number-10: 0-309-08870-4
Digital Object Identifier: https://doi.org/10.17226/26284
Library of Congress Catalog Number: 2021951345

Additional copies of this publication are available from the National Academies Press, 500 Fifth Street, NW, Keck 360, Washington, DC 20001; (800) 624-6242 or (202) 334-3313; http://www.nap.edu.

Printed in the United States of America

Suggested citation: National Academies of Sciences, Engineering, and Medicine. 2022. *Countering the pandemic threat through global coordination on vaccines: The influenza imperative.* Washington, DC: The National Academies Press. https://doi.org/10.17226/26284.

The National Academies of

SCIENCES • ENGINEERING • MEDICINE

The **National Academy of Sciences** was established in 1863 by an Act of Congress, signed by President Lincoln, as a private, nongovernmental institution to advise the nation on issues related to science and technology. Members are elected by their peers for outstanding contributions to research. Dr. Marcia McNutt is president.

The **National Academy of Engineering** was established in 1964 under the charter of the National Academy of Sciences to bring the practices of engineering to advising the nation. Members are elected by their peers for extraordinary contributions to engineering. Dr. John L. Anderson is president.

The **National Academy of Medicine** (formerly the Institute of Medicine) was established in 1970 under the charter of the National Academy of Sciences to advise the nation on medical and health issues. Members are elected by their peers for distinguished contributions to medicine and health. Dr. Victor J. Dzau is president.

The three Academies work together as the **National Academies of Sciences, Engineering, and Medicine** to provide independent, objective analysis and advice to the nation and conduct other activities to solve complex problems and inform public policy decisions. The National Academies also encourage education and research, recognize outstanding contributions to knowledge, and increase public understanding in matters of science, engineering, and medicine.

Learn more about the National Academies of Sciences, Engineering, and Medicine at **www.nationalacademies.org.**

The National Academies of
SCIENCES · ENGINEERING · MEDICINE

COMMITTEE ON GLOBAL COORDINATION, PARTNERSHIPS, AND FINANCING RECOMMENDATIONS FOR ADVANCING PANDEMIC AND SEASONAL INFLUENZA VACCINE PREPAREDNESS AND RESPONSE

PETER SANDS (*Chair*), Executive Director, The Global Fund to Fight AIDS, Tuberculosis and Malaria
DEVI SRIDHAR (*Vice Chair*), Professor and Chair of Global Public Health, Usher Institute, University of Edinburgh
SALAH T. AL AWAIDY, Communicable Disease Advisor, Ministry of Health, Oman
WILLIAM AMPOFO, Associate Professor, Virology Department, Noguchi Memorial Institute for Medical Research, University of Ghana
PHYLLIS ARTHUR, Vice President, Infectious Diseases and Emerging Science Policy, Biotechnology Innovation Organization
CHRISTOPHER T. BAUCH, Professor of Applied Mathematics, University of Waterloo
GIAN LUCA BURCI, Professor of International Law, Graduate Institute of International and Development Studies
KEIJI FUKUDA, Director and Clinical Professor, School of Public Health, LKS Faculty of Medicine, The University of Hong Kong
BRUCE G. GELLIN, Chief, Global Public Health Strategy, The Rockefeller Foundation
AMANDA L. GLASSMAN, Executive Vice President and Senior Fellow, Center for Global Development
RICHARD J. HATCHETT, Chief Executive Officer, Coalition for Epidemic Preparedness Innovations
JOHN NKENGASONG, Director, Africa Centres for Disease Control and Prevention
CHARLES "OK" PANNENBORG, Chief Health Scientist and Director, World Bank (Retired)
ALEXANDRA L. PHELAN, Assistant Professor, Center for Global Health Science and Security, Georgetown University Medical Center, Adjunct Professor, Georgetown University Law Center
CHRISTOPHER SNYDER, Joel and Susan Hyatt Professor of Economics, Department of Economics, Dartmouth College
CHARLOTTE WELLER, Head of Prevention, Wellcome Trust

Study Staff

JANELLE WINTERS, Study Director
CLAIRE MOERDER, Research Associate (*until June 2021*)

ERIKA JAUREGUI, Research Associate (*from June to August 2021*)
INEZ ADAMS, Research Associate (*from June to August 2021*)
TOCHI OGBU-MBADIUGHA, Senior Program Assistant (*from April 2021*)
EMILIE RYAN-CASTILLO, Senior Program Assistant
PATRICIA A. CUFF, Senior Program Officer, Board on Global Health
JULIE A. PAVLIN, Senior Director, Board on Global Health
FRANCES SHARPLES, Science Writer
ROGER YAT-NORK CHUNG, National Academy of Medicine International Health Policy Fellow

Consultant

ANNA NICHOLSON, Science Writer

Reviewers

This Consensus Study Report was reviewed in draft form by individuals chosen for their diverse perspectives and technical expertise. The purpose of this independent review is to provide candid and critical comments that will assist the National Academies of Sciences, Engineering, and Medicine in making each published report as sound as possible and to ensure that it meets the institutional standards for quality, objectivity, evidence, and responsiveness to the study charge. The review comments and draft manuscript remain confidential to protect the integrity of the deliberative process.

We thank the following individuals for their review of this report:

SUSAN ATHEY, Stanford Institute for Economic Policy Research
CARLOS CORREA, South Centre
MARK DYBUL, Georgetown University Medical Center
DAVID FIDLER, Council on Foreign Relations
KEITH KLUGMAN, Bill & Melinda Gates Foundation
ANUP MALANI, University of Chicago Law School
DEEPALI PATEL, Gavi, the Vaccine Alliance
SAI D. PRASAD, Bharat Biotech International Ltd.
NITEEN WAIRAGKAR, Vaccines for All

Although the reviewers listed above provided many constructive comments and suggestions, they were not asked to endorse the conclusions or recommendations of this report, nor did they see the final draft before its release. The review of this report was overseen by **GAIL CASSELL,**

Harvard University, and **HELEN MILNER,** Princeton University. They were responsible for making certain that an independent examination of this report was carried out in accordance with the standards of the National Academies and that all review comments were carefully considered. Responsibility for the final content rests entirely with the authoring committee and the National Academies.

National Academy of Medicine

Advancing Pandemic and Seasonal Influenza Vaccine Preparedness and Response Series

This study, Countering the Pandemic Threat Through Global Coordination on Vaccines: The Influenza Imperative, provides recommendations on how to identify and overcome barriers to effective global coordination and sustainable financing for pandemic and seasonal influenza vaccines and vaccinations, drawing on successes and challenges from the global response to COVID-19. It is one of four studies conducted under the Advancing Pandemic and Seasonal Influenza Vaccine Preparedness and Response Initiative, which explores how the scientific and technological breakthroughs throughout the COVID-19 pandemic could inform and advance future pandemic and seasonal influenza vaccine preparedness and response efforts.

The three companion studies to this study examine how the lessons learned from COVID-19 around vaccine research and development, vaccine distribution and supply chain, and public health interventions and countermeasures could be best utilized to improve the development and distribution of future pandemic and seasonal influenza vaccines. Together, the four consensus studies present a path toward better preparedness in addressing pandemic and seasonal influenza.

Launched by the National Academy of Medicine with support from the Office of Global Affairs, U.S. Department of Health and Human Services, the Advancing Pandemic and Seasonal Influenza Vaccine Preparedness and Response Initiative acknowledges that influenza is here to stay. The unprecedented scope of this initiative allowed for international experts to look at this issue from multiple angles and provide recommendations that set out a pathway to more effective influenza vaccines worldwide. Driven by international cooperation, this independent initiative provides a platform to highlight why we need to act as a global community to better prepare for pandemic and seasonal influenza.

Acknowledgments

This study is timely, in terms of considering how to harness lessons and best prepare for a major future pandemic threat during a debilitating current pandemic. This timeliness created an intense study schedule for the committee members and staff. First and foremost, we would like to thank the members of the pandemic preparedness and response (PPR) community who took the time to speak to us, on top of *incredibly* busy schedules. Appendix B lists the names and affiliations of all speakers. This study would not have been possible without their intellectual contributions and candid perspectives on what has worked (and not worked) in pandemic preparedness for COVID-19, influenza, and other threats. We would also like to thank our sponsor, the Office of Global Affairs in the U.S. Department of Health and Human Services. We appreciate your dedication to advancing the pandemic influenza preparedness agenda. We are further indebted to members of the influenza PPR international committee, under the umbrella of the National Academy of Medicine, who guided the development of the four consensus studies. Finally, we thank members of the Health and Medicine Division, particularly Lauren Shern for providing study guidance and Leslie Sim and Taryn Young for coordinating the review process. Last, but certainly not least, we are grateful for the support of members of the "flu team" at the Board on Global Health, especially Kenisha Jefferson, Ellen Schenk, and Hoda Soltani.

Preface

COVID-19 has taught the world a harsh lesson on the perils of being unprepared for a pandemic. More than 18 months since the World Health Organization (WHO) declared a public health emergency of international concern, governments across the world are still struggling to contain new waves of infection and death. The human and economic costs of this crisis are staggering, and it is far from over.

This reality underscores this report's title, *Countering the Pandemic Threat Through Global Coordination on Vaccines: The Influenza Imperative.* COVID-19 has been terrible, but an *influenza* pandemic comparable to that of 1918–1919 could be even worse. The world cannot afford to be as unprepared for an influenza pandemic as we turned out to be for COVID-19. So, while the immediate priority must be to defeat COVID-19, we must also move decisively to strengthen our ability to protect people from future threats, pandemic influenza above all.

The seven recommendations in this report aim to provide this agenda for action. Underpinning the recommendations are four crosscutting themes. The first is simply the inadequacy of our current defenses: we have too many gaps, and too much is dependent on underfunded, often informal arrangements. Against the scale of the threat, we are woefully underprotected. We urgently need to strengthen our collective defenses against pandemic influenza and must do so in a way that is sustainable.

The second theme is the need to integrate the solutions for pandemic influenza into whatever broader solution global policy makers devise for pandemic preparedness and response (PPR) through the G7 or G20. It no longer makes sense to have purely influenza-specific mechanisms for critical capabilities, such as disease surveillance, pathogen sharing, vaccine platform technologies, and vaccine deployment systems. The G7 and G20 debates around determining this broader set of solutions have been unfolding in parallel with the committee's deliberations, posing a challenge in framing our recommendations: we want our proposals for pandemic influenza to fit the broader overarching solution for pandemic preparedness, without yet knowing precisely what this will look like.

The third theme is in slight tension with the second. We must integrate influenza PPR with the broader pandemic preparedness agenda, but we must avoid inadvertently weakening the existing influenza mechanisms. For all their limitations, current arrangements for global coordination, partnerships, and financing for pandemic influenza are typically much more established than the equivalents for other pathogens of pandemic potential. Moreover, influenza's unique characteristics, such as its seasonality, create distinct challenges and opportunities that must be factored into the preparedness approach.

The fourth and final theme revolves around equity. Unless equity is embedded into the mechanisms for influenza PPR, frictions about inequitable access will corrode the collaboration and partnerships that are so vital to protecting us all. Moral, epidemiological, and practical perspectives all point to the need for an equitable approach to PPR.

The world might be lucky and not face an influenza pandemic for decades. But we might also be unlucky and find ourselves confronted by such a threat even before we surmount COVID-19. We cannot rely on luck. Too much is at stake. More effective global coordination, deeper partnerships, and scaled-up and sustained financing are essential to deliver reinforced protection against pandemic influenza. This committee, combining in its membership an extraordinary range of experience and expertise, aided by the superb staff of the National Academies, and informed by exceptional speakers bringing a wide spectrum of perspectives, has sought to explore these issues and lay out a set of actionable recommendations to address this imperative and make us all safer from the threat of pandemic influenza.

Peter Sands, *Chair*
Committee on Global Coordination, Partnerships, and
Financing Recommendations for Advancing Pandemic and
Seasonal Influenza Vaccine Preparedness and Response

Contents

Boxes, Figures, and Tables

BOXES

FIGURES

TABLES

Acronyms and Abbreviations

ABS	access and benefit sharing
Africa CDC	Africa Centres for Disease Control and Prevention
AMC	advance market commitment
AU	African Union
BARDA	Biomedical Advanced Research and Development Authority
BMGF	Bill & Melinda Gates Foundation
CBD	Convention on Biological Diversity
CC	WHO Collaborating Center
CDC	U.S. Centers for Disease Control and Prevention
CEPI	Coalition for Epidemic Preparedness Innovations
CIDRAP	Center for Infectious Disease Research and Policy
COVAX	COVID-19 Vaccines Global Access
CRS	U.S. Congressional Research Service
CVV	candidate vaccine virus
DARPA	Defense Advanced Research Project Agency
EU	European Union
FAO	Food and Agriculture Organization of the United Nations

FCTC	Framework Convention on Tobacco Control
GAO	U.S. Government Accountability Office
GAP	WHO Global Vaccine Action Plan
GIP	Global Influenza Program
GISN	Global Influenza Surveillance Network
GISRS	Global Influenza Surveillance and Response System
GLEWS	Global Early Warning System for Major Animal Diseases
GloPID-R	Global Research Collaboration for Infectious Disease Preparedness
GPMB	Global Preparedness Monitoring Board
HERA	Health Emergency Preparedness and Response Authority Incubator
HIC	high-income country
HLIP	G20 High-Level Independent Panel on Financing the Global Commons for Pandemic Preparedness and Response
IFC	International Finance Corporation
IFPMA	International Federation of Pharmaceutical Manufacturers & Associations
IHR	International Health Regulations
IIV	inactivated influenza vaccines
IMF	International Monetary Fund
IP	intellectual property
IPPPR	Independent Panel for Pandemic Preparedness and Response
IVPP	influenza viruses with pandemic potential
LAIV	live attenuated influenza vaccine
LMIC	low- and middle-income country
MERS	Middle East respiratory syndrome
MIT	Massachusetts Institute of Technology
mRNA	messenger RNA
NGO	nongovernmental organization
NIAID	National Institute of Allergy and Infectious Diseases
NIC	WHO National Influenza Centre

OECD	Organisation for Economic Co-operation and Development
OFFLU	OIE/FAO Joint Network of Expertise on Animal Influenza
OIE	World Organisation for Animal Health
OWS	Operation Warp Speed
PHEIC	Public Health Emergency of International Concern
PIP	Pandemic Influenza Preparedness Framework
PPP	G7/UK International Pandemic Preparedness Partnership
PPR	pandemic preparedness and response
R&D	research and development
REDISSE	World Bank Regional Disease Surveillance Systems Enhancement Project in West Africa
SARS	severe acute respiratory syndrome
SMTA-2	standard material transfer agreement 2
TAG	technical advisory group
TWN	Third World Network
UNICEF	United Nations Children's Fund
WHA	World Health Assembly
WHO	World Health Organization
WTO	World Trade Organization

Summary

As of October 6, 2021, the global number of cases of COVID-19 had surpassed 235 million, with deaths approaching 5 million worldwide.[1] These figures are likely to be substantial underestimates. For example, a July 2021 study from the Center for Global Development (Anand et al., 2021) provided an analysis of death numbers for India that suggested that the toll of 400,000 underestimated the true number by a factor of 10. Furthermore, in June 2021, economists estimated that the pandemic led to a 6.65 percent loss of global gross domestic product (GDP) in 2020 alone. COVID-19 is also likely to have lasting effects on global GDP due to the costs of fiscal stimuli, the value of excess deaths, and other factors, such as the loss of businesses and educational opportunities. These effects may lead to a 54.68 percent loss of total GDP from 2020 to 2030 (Yeyati and Filippini, 2021).

Yet, from an epidemiological perspective, COVID-19 does not represent a "worst-case" pandemic scenario, such as the 1918–1919 influenza, which resulted in at least 50 million deaths worldwide (Taubenberger and Morens, 2006). Influenza pandemics have occurred repeatedly, and experts worry that the risk for an influenza pandemic may be even higher during the COVID-19 era due to changes in global and regional conditions affecting humans, animals, and their contact patterns. While it is difficult to predict when it will occur, a major influenza pandemic is more a matter of "when" than "if" (Kelland, 2019).

Although the true burden of influenza is unknown, an estimated 1 billion people are infected by seasonal influenza annually and in virtually

[1] See Johns Hopkins Coronavirus Resource Center, https://coronavirus.jhu.edu.

every country (WHO, 2019a). This affects almost an eighth of the world's population every year (Palache et al., 2020). Among the large family of influenza viruses, a subgroup that predominately infects mammalian animals and birds are considered potential pandemic strains. Similar to the viruses that have caused severe acute respiratory syndrome (SARS) and COVID-19, certain novel influenza A viruses might have the capability and opportunity to make the jump from animals to become highly infectious for humans and so cause a pandemic. Influenza pandemics are a serious threat, and, because of their respiratory mode of transmission and short incubation period, they are capable of spreading rapidly around the world and causing high illness and death. Yet, the public and policy makers are mainly only familiar with seasonal influenza and, paradoxically, often dismiss *all* influenza and a range of minor illnesses with similar symptoms as "just the flu." To place the threat of pandemic influenza in context, if COVID-19 had the same case fatality rate as the 1918–1919 influenza, the total U.S. death toll alone would approach 2 million[2] (Ewing, 2021). A pandemic caused by a novel influenza strain of moderate to severe lethality would likely cost the modern world economy trillions of dollars (GPMB, 2019).

The year 2020 saw unprecedented innovation and scientific collaboration related to vaccine research and development, with special attention on the decades of work to develop messenger RNA (mRNA) technology and other rapid response platforms that were ready for and applied to produce highly effective vaccines for COVID-19. Three to four times more COVID-19 vaccine, almost 12 billion doses, are projected to be available by the end of 2021, compared to what was possible for *all vaccines* in 2019 (IFPMA, 2021). If we were experiencing pandemic influenza instead, would global stakeholders have been willing at the outset to embrace the newer, barely tested vaccine technologies, or would they have stayed with the familiar and well-tested largely egg-based approaches? According to 2019 estimates, if everything went right, 6.4 billion influenza vaccine doses could theoretically have been produced over 12 months, using mostly egg-based technologies (Sparrow et al., 2021). Based on commitments from industrial partners to the World Health Organization (WHO) Pandemic Influenza Preparedness (PIP) Framework, only about 400 million doses of pandemic vaccine would have been available for WHO to distribute globally during that period. The reliance on largely egg-based technologies and the use of adjuvants (both of which have limited surge capacity) highlights the need for the world to be much better prepared to make and distribute vaccines to counter an influenza pandemic.

---

[2] As of October 6, 2021, the confirmed U.S. death toll from COVID-19 was 705,404 according to data from the Johns Hopkins Coronavirus Resource Center, https://coronavirus.jhu.edu (accessed October 6, 2021).

The enormous innovations in vaccine development and production that emerged for COVID-19—supported by many new public–private partnerships (PPPs)—suggest technological options for making greater quantities of influenza vaccines more quickly. Much research and development (R&D) needs to be done to establish the general applicability of these new approaches to developing and manufacturing vaccines for influenza and other pathogens. For these technologies and platforms to be available and scaled up when the world needs them, workforce, regulatory capacity, and business models must also be in place. Readiness to respond to a pandemic requires a corresponding increase in the use of these facilities between pandemics. This increased usage is critical for reducing the impact of seasonal influenza but will also help ensure that manufacturing facilities stay operational between pandemics.

The COVID-19 pandemic has laid bare the "fragility of our global system of preparedness and response to pandemics, and the fragmentation of our research and development ecosystem" (Lurie et al., 2021). It also provides a disruptive moment to significantly act on pandemic preparedness and response (PPR)—including advancing new norms and frameworks for influenza. How should influenza fit within the wider PPR agenda, which is currently being advanced by the G7 via the UK Pandemic Preparedness Partnership and the G20 through its High-Level Independent Panel (HLIP) on Financing the Global Commons for Pandemic Preparedness and Response? What governance frameworks and regulations need to be safeguarded around influenza specifically, and what should be expanded from influenza to other respiratory pathogens with pandemic potential?

With these questions in mind, an ad hoc committee of experts was formed under the auspices of the National Academies of Sciences, Engineering, and Medicine (the National Academies) and tasked to examine recent experiences during COVID-19 and other major viral epidemics and identify ways to strengthen pandemic and seasonal influenza global coordination, partnerships, and financing. The committee's deliberations were based on a single premise: starting with the first human detection of a novel influenza virus with pandemic potential, how can the global health community move as quickly as possible to develop and produce safe and effective vaccines and equitably immunize as many people as possible worldwide? The committee acknowledges that a universal influenza vaccine would be a complete game changer, by ensuring advance preparation rather than reactive development. The report's chapters encompass the governance and financing structures required to support rapid developments to vaccination at scale, including surveillance, pathogen sharing, partnerships for technology (R&D and vaccine optimization) and manufacturing (vaccine scale-up and manufacturing facilities), and access and financing (financing mechanisms to "push" and "pull," procure, and nationally deploy influenza vaccines). Based on its findings and conclusions, the committee draws seven overarching recommendations for how the urgent influenza threat should be conceptualized and prioritized as a crucial component of the broader global PPR agenda over the next 3–5 years.

The committee further acknowledges that its recommendations presume a degree of cohesion and commitment to a global common purpose across the G7 and G20, which cannot be taken for granted, despite the compelling economic and human case for collective action to reinforce PPR. The changing dynamics of international relations over the past decade or so have transformed the geopolitical context in which global health policy is made. Shifts in the balance of power in the international system; the rise of authoritarian states; diminished cohesion of democratic states; and the rise of nationalism and populism across a broad array of states are among the factors that have led to this transformation. The COVID-19 response has exposed sharp fissures in the international order, shaking confidence in the notion of a global community and revealing the powerful, complex, and somewhat contradictory interactions between global health priorities, domestic political imperatives, and other dimensions of geopolitical competition and collaboration. Major powers in the G7 and G20 have simultaneously supported efforts to promote equitable access to vaccines and actively engaged in "vaccine nationalism." Meanwhile, "vaccine diplomacy" has been used to garner geopolitical and ideological advantage. One of the biggest and most sobering lessons from COVID-19 has been that in an infectious disease crisis of this magnitude, neither established arrangements, such as the International Health Regulations (IHR 2005) nor newly created mechanisms, such as COVAX, can withstand the overwhelming pressures to prioritize national interests.

The committee did not directly consider how to address these daunting geopolitical challenges, as doing so would involve venturing far beyond its mandate. However, the committee recognizes that overcoming these challenges, or at least mitigating their consequences for global health, is a prerequisite for success, for both the broader PPR agenda and the specific influenza vaccine recommendations that this committee put forward. The committee adopted the basic assumption that a geopolitical context can be established in which one can speak meaningfully of a global community able to take at least some degree of coordinated collective action, since much of what is proposed in the recommendations requires this as a foundation. This does not require global consensus on everything or mean that every country is involved in every effort, but it implies a base level of coordination among leading states. As a shorthand expression and recognizing that this is an imperfect depiction of the stakeholders involved, this report typically refers to the G7 and G20 as the nexus of such a global community.

The committee also recognizes that it is possible to construct some technical coordination mechanisms in a "flying under the radar" mode that is somewhat insulated from politics. However, the committee is skeptical about relying too much on such an approach. COVID-19 has repeatedly revealed how the intense political pressures that arise from a deadly pandemic can override technical, contractual, or legal considerations. As the G7 and G20 devise a new set of mechanisms to bolster PPR, including potentially new legal obligations (e.g., from a pandemic treaty or instrument, should this emerge), new governance arrangements (such as a Global Health Threats Board), and new means for financing (such as HLIP's proposal of a Global Health Threats Fund), it is important to recognize that when put to the test, these new arrangements are unlikely to work precisely as designed because national interests will once again prove almost impossible to withstand. But recognizing their limitations does not equate to believing that such arrangements have no value: they can be enormously helpful in shifting norms and behaviors, such as toward more equitable deployment of lifesaving medical tools.

KEY FINDINGS AND RECOMMENDATIONS

Governance and Coordination: Aligned Pandemic Preparedness and Response for Respiratory Pathogens with Pandemic Potential

Among infectious diseases with pandemic potential, influenza stands out because its technical and policy systems, including for surveillance, the vaccine strain selection process, relations between the public and private sectors, and related access and benefit system (pertaining to pandemic influenza) are global and—at least compared to other pathogens—relatively well coordinated through WHO. These pre-existing arrangements constitute a functional, if limited, "ecosystem" to address seasonal and pandemic influenza. Despite many aspects of these mechanisms that need substantial strengthening, the starting point for influenza is very different from other pathogens of pandemic potential. The COVID-19 pandemic led to a wide recognition of the need to reinforce PPR for the various pathogens potentially capable of causing a pandemic. A pressing need exists to integrate actions to strengthen preparedness for pandemic influenza with interventions to improve it for other pathogens, particularly other respiratory viruses. Without undermining what is already in place, it is necessary to move away from disease-specific, siloed systems toward developing an integrated governance, financing, technical, and operational architecture capable of addressing all respiratory virus pandemic threats. An example in this direction related to surveillance would be the Global Influenza Surveillance and Response System "plus" (GISRS+) proposal.

Recommendation 1: The World Health Organization (WHO) should develop an integrated agenda to strengthen preparedness and response for all respiratory pathogens of pandemic potential, which includes surveillance, information sharing, and the development, manufacturing, and deployment of vaccines and other essential components of the vaccine manufacturing supply chain. This agenda should comprise a key component of the overarching agenda for pandemic preparedness and response, encompass pandemic influenza, and build on existing mechanisms for coordination in the influenza arena. To accomplish this, member states should task WHO to:

a. Assume leadership for this agenda and, with collaboration from relevant multilateral partners (e.g., the Food and Agriculture Organization of the United Nations and the World Organisation for Animal Health), propose a framework for strengthened surveillance systems and information sharing at country, regional, and global levels to ensure rapid detection of new threats and enable swift dissemination of information essential to accelerated vaccine development.
b. Work jointly with existing international and stakeholder organizations with expertise in vaccine research and development, manufacturing coordination and supply chain management, and deployment (e.g., the Coalition for Epidemic Preparedness Innovations, the United Nations Children's Fund, and Gavi, the Vaccine Alliance) to develop, in consultation with vaccine manufacturers, a framework for improved global coordination of vaccine development, production, and deployment for respiratory pathogens with pandemic potential that includes defined roles, responsibilities, and accountability mechanisms.

Surveillance: Stable Financing for Integrated, Modern, Timely Respiratory Virus Surveillance for Pathogens with Pandemic Potential

Without stable financing of a modern, integrated surveillance system for respiratory pathogens with pandemic potential, we will continue to fight pandemics in the dark. In the information era, the lack of reliable, sustained, and globally connected systems is striking and has massive negative ramifications for national, regional, and global health security. Surveillance system gaps reflect insufficient financing and political will, and top to bottom attention will be needed to build, more closely align, and integrate such systems. This is not a low- and middle-income country (LMIC) problem only; many high-income countries (HICs) have moved away from adequately financing surveillance systems, and many systems underperform in terms of rapidly identifying, assessing, and reporting potential threats.

Moreover, the known science of pandemic threats indicates that effective surveillance systems must work across traditional sector silos, including human and animal health and agriculture, to identify and assess zoonotic threats and spillover events and rapidly disseminate the data and insights that these yield. Establishing and sustaining broader surveillance systems has been challenged by both scientific and cultural silos, including how to cover multiple pathogens in an integrated system, because certain aspects may differ greatly (e.g., different scientific expertise and specimen collection requirements). However, all pathogens have significant commonalities (e.g., standardized data and systems), and an integrated approach to risk assessments would benefit from the efficiencies of shared platforms and approaches.

Strengthening and broadening global influenza surveillance to support a broader approach to respiratory virus surveillance will require substantially greater and sustained multilateral investments in country, regional, and global surveillance. Surveillance is primarily a global and national risk assessment and mitigation issue. Each country's surveillance system generates significant positive externalities (benefits that accrue to other countries). This also provides a strong argument for external financing for surveillance when domestic resources are inadequate.

The Independent Panel for Pandemic Preparedness and Response (IPPPR) and other groups are working on recommendations for institutional mechanisms for surveillance, including for a global viral surveillance network. This committee's findings and deliberations underscore that integrated viral surveillance should be structured to support country ownership and cover critical *influenza* data needs as an integrated system, including genomic sequences, specimens for testing, and viruses from both human and animal sources. Surveillance must be viewed as an essential foundation for preventing and responding to threats rapidly and effectively by furnishing information essential for developing medical countermeasures. Enhancing such systems to monitor and assess a range of pandemic threats, including influenza and as-yet-unknown threats, will require a dedicated, sustained pool of financing at national, regional, and global levels that must be sustained, stable, and long term.

Recommendation 2: With urgency (over the next 3–5 years), the G7 and G20 should ensure that increased investments are made in surveillance systems for pathogens with pandemic potential, which support and encompass every country and region, by doing the following:

a. **Creating incentives, structures, and pathways for key stakeholders to develop and implement integrated surveillance, which should include firmer support for zoonotic surveillance in the framework of One Health programs, such as through the World Health Organization (WHO), the World Organisation** for Animal Health (OIE), and the Food and Agriculture Organization of the United Nations (FAO) stakeholders.

b. Strengthening and financing regional surveillance structures and networks through partnerships between regional development banks and organizations. For example, in the South Asia and Southeast Asia regions this could be accomplished in conjunction with the Association of Southeast Asian Nations, Asian Development Bank, and Asian Infrastructure Investment Bank, and in the Middle East and North Africa with the Organization of Islamic Cooperation, Gulf Cooperation Council, and Islamic Development Bank.
c. Ensuring that the financing mechanism selected by the G7/G20 for pandemic preparedness and response more broadly includes sustainable funding for surveillance and that this pooled funding is sufficient to enable surveillance for respiratory pathogens, especially encompassing those with pandemic potential, at the national and regional levels.
d. This global funding mechanism's governance should include relevant international agencies, such as the International Fund for Agricultural Development, OIE, FAO, and the World Food Program, in addition to multilateral and regional development banks and WHO.

Pathogen Sharing: Limitations and Potential of the PIP Framework and Nagoya Protocol

The timely sharing of influenza viruses is essential for developing life-saving seasonal influenza vaccines, identifying antiviral drug resistance and potential pandemic virus strains, and providing early warning for outbreaks. The PIP Framework supports a critical WHO global surveillance system needed for influenza and establishes a multilateral agreement that places access and benefit sharing (ABS) and sharing of viruses of pandemic potential on an equal footing but avoids a bilateral transactional approach to such sharing. It reflects the importance of transparency, equity, efficiency, and the accountability shared by countries, industry, and WHO.

If a new global pandemic treaty or international instrument is negotiated (see Chapter 3), it will provide an opportunity to incorporate and consolidate diplomatic gains from the earlier PIP Framework negotiations and agreements as foundational elements for new multilateral solutions. Having such a multilateral instrument could eliminate the challenge of negotiating the sharing of viruses and benefits in the midst of a pandemic, ensuring greater predictability, and saving critical time and attention needed during a full response. The principles agreed upon in the

PIP Framework could be incorporated into the foundations of any future pandemic instrument.

Seasonal pathogen sharing has increasingly been negatively impacted by the Nagoya Protocol, resulting in the need in some instances to choose alternate virus strains for vaccines (WHO, 2019b). In a pandemic, delays in sharing viruses and associated information could have very serious implications for delaying the response. A similar delay in sharing genetic sequence data is also possible, due to the uncertainty about whether it falls under the PIP Framework and Nagoya Protocol. The rapid ramp-up of genomic surveillance for SARS-CoV-2 variants and the use of such data for vaccine development underscores the urgency of ensuring rapid access and sharing of genetic sequence data during pandemic situations.

Recommendation 3: The World Health Assembly (WHA) should explicitly clarify that the Pandemic Influenza Preparedness (PIP) Framework covers genetic sequence data. The WHA should also use established PIP Framework principles as a foundation for future World Health Organization (WHO) member state agreements, or advocate for their use in agreements negotiated by other international organizations, so that the access and benefit and information-sharing principles cover a broader range of pathogens and their genetic sequence data. To accomplish this, the WHA should, with support of the United Nations, do the following:

a. **Establish accountability and compliance monitoring for member states and other parties in the PIP Framework and future agreements on access and benefit sharing (ABS) through regular reviews and meetings of member states, and by building or strengthening norms and holding leaders accountable for following through on commitments.**
b. **Incorporate the principles of equity, shared accountability, and multilateralism in any future pandemic treaty or instrument and ensure that the surveillance systems that can rapidly detect, assess, report, and share these viruses are publicly recognized to be a global public good.**
c. **Develop a mechanism for countries to share viruses openly and rapidly, including their genetic sequences and other essential supporting laboratory information and epidemiological data for both risk assessment and risk management (developing vaccines, therapeutics, and diagnostics), while setting up incentives for industry and member states to share benefits and products (vaccines, therapeutics, and diagnostics), and to facilitate transferring technology. This requires a recognition of the concerns of industry over intellectual property. This mechanism should**

include regular public reporting as part of a transparency and monitoring system to hold countries and governments accountable for their level of pandemic preparedness and response.

d. Request that the WHO secretariat approach the Convention on Biological Diversity (CBD) secretariat to initiate a process for a new international agreement or instrument to be established as a "special international instrument" under Article 4.4 of the Nagoya Protocol (allowing the agreement to bypass some Nagoya Protocol requirements while remaining consistent with its objectives). The new international agreement or instrument could either be negotiated as an additional protocol to the CBD alongside the Nagoya Protocol, be a component of a possible future pandemic treaty, or be negotiated within WHO as a new ad hoc international agreement. The special international instrument should address the sharing of genetic sequence data and other necessary information, such as important epidemiological and laboratory data, in addition to the pathogen samples. The Meeting of the Parties to the Nagoya Protocol, in collaboration with WHO, should recommend that Parties to the Protocol facilitate and streamline national implementation procedures to facilitate the timely international sharing of pathogens in line with the urgency of responding to an outbreak. The Meeting should also acknowledge that genetic sequences of both human and animal pathogens are essential for modern science to adequately assess and respond to outbreak emergencies and to develop optimal vaccines, diagnostic tests, and other critical materials. Consideration should also be given to reinforcing that any ABS portion of the agreement not deter innovation or act as a disincentive for industry participation.

Public–Private Partnerships to Accelerate Vaccine Development: Structuring Global Partnerships to Support R&D for Influenza Platform Technologies

PPPs with industry before and during the COVID-19 pandemic have allowed highly efficacious platform technology–based vaccines to be developed. Platform technologies could revolutionize the effectiveness, speed, and ability to scale up production of influenza vaccines and overcome some intrinsic constraints of the current egg-dominated ecosystem. This establishes a *necessity of innovation* for influenza vaccines to shorten manufacturing time lines, increase global manufacturing capacity, and improve effectiveness. The goal in the next 3–5 years would be to progressively pursue development and assessment of new platform technologies to improve vaccine effectiveness, expand the options for scalability and production, and optimize their methods, in parallel to pursuing the "ultimate prize," a universal influenza vaccine (see Recommendation 5). As highlighted by the Center for Infectious Disease Research and Policy (CIDRAP) Influenza Vaccine Roadmap, because of influenza's high mutation rate and other characteristics, this will require significant investment in early R&D, including support of Phase I–III clinical trials and vaccine dose optimization. It will also require recognizing intellectual property issues, to foster a continued willingness of industry to form synergistic partnerships.

The difficulty is in how to scale up industry partnerships and apply them globally, especially to support a geographically distributed manufacturing hub model. Several existing organizations (Coalition for Epidemic Preparedness Innovations [CEPI], Biomedical Advanced Research and Development Authority [BARDA], and the new HERA Incubator) may be able to lead large-scale R&D and clinical trials for influenza platform technologies, including large-scale global action in LMICs, if they are given expanded mandates matched with appropriate funding and can identify stable markets for their products.

As a PPP with a multilateral approach, CEPI is well positioned to address the coordination and cost-effectiveness challenges for influenza R&D on a global scale. However, BARDA and HERA have similar capacities for advanced vaccine development, at the early, middle, and late stages. Giving BARDA a broader remit may allow it to overcome a limitation of Operation Warp Speed (OWS): that it only focused on U.S. needs and did not account for global needs or engage with a broader set of global stakeholders and partners.[3]

Recommendation 4: The Global Health Threats Board or similar governance structure created by the G7/G20 PPR agenda, should negotiate to extend the mandates of the Coalition for Epidemic Preparedness Innovations (CEPI), the Biomedical Advanced Research and Development Authority, the HERA Incubator, and equivalents elsewhere as appropriate, to support government–industry partnerships for research and development (R&D) for influenza and other respiratory viruses with pandemic potential. These voluntary partnerships should focus

[3] The committee wishes to highlight that its membership includes Richard Hatchett, the chief executive officer of CEPI, and Charlotte Weller, head of Prevention at the Wellcome Trust, who chairs the CEPI Investors Council in a voluntary capacity. Recommendations 4 and 5 include actions in which CEPI could play a significant role. These recommendations are based on a consensus from all committee members based on the evidence available.

on optimizing each industry partner's platform, using the following structure:

a. The G7 and G20 member nations (e.g., through the Global Health Threats Board) should name a global coordination body to specifically coordinate global and regional government–industry partnerships for influenza vaccines. CEPI is the existing multilateral global coordination vehicle for R&D, has access principles built in, and is a possible organization to assume this role.
b. Countries that fund vaccine R&D should ensure that R&D for pandemic influenza is part of their funding portfolio and strive to identify investment synergies to maximize returns on investments. Regional organizations should support the mobilization of government–industry partnerships, such as the Africa Centres for Disease Control and Prevention, the Association of Southeast Asian Nations, the Gulf Cooperation Council, and Europe 2020's Innovation Union (funded by HORIZON 2020) and its successor.
c. Government–industry partnerships should have affiliated teams to identify promising technologies, optimize them for the field (e.g., identify adjuvants that enhance vaccine products on a small scale, to provide directionality in what to do during a surge), and consider investments required to reach efficiency yields. These partnerships should support Phase I–III clinical trials, as recommended by the United Kingdom/G7 Independent Panel for Pandemic Preparedness and Response, as well as early dosing trials. They should also build in workforce development training for areas of expertise required to be "at the table" for technology transfer of these products.
d. Government–industry partnerships should share workforce development requirements with CEPI, the World Health Organization, and other relevant multilateral partners, to help countries identify and fill gaps in ministries of health, labor, and economics expertise before a pandemic.

An Influenza Vaccine Moonshot: Financing and Organizing for Transformational Universal Vaccine R&D, Licensure, and Procurement

Seasonal influenza vaccines are reformulated annually to target the viral antigens that are anticipated to circulate in the northern and southern hemispheres that year. Influenza can also develop significant mutations (genetic shift) and present a pandemic virus for which there is no existing population immunity. A universal influenza vaccine would, in theory, be able to induce immunity against most or all influenza A virus strains, including future pandemic strains. The availability of such a vaccine is the subject of ongoing research and would be a significant game changer for both pandemic and seasonal influenza preparedness and response and vaccine markets. Developing such a vaccine remains a difficult scientific problem with no guarantee that a vaccine can be developed that will provide long-term protection in people of all age groups. However, a universal influenza vaccine would be transformational.

Developing improved influenza vaccine technologies will require major intensification of fundamental and applied research. Substantive new sources of funding are needed to attract an infusion of new actors and new disciplines (e.g., computational and systems biology, bioinformatics, artificial intelligence, deep learning, machine learning, and HIV/AIDS and cancer immunotherapy research communities) (BMGF, 2021). Push incentives will be critical to fully enable cross-disciplinary problem solving and achieve and demonstrate a proof of concept, while pull incentives, such as advance market commitments (AMCs), will be needed for sustainability of a commercial product in the influenza vaccine market. Kremer and Glennerster (2004) originally proposed the AMC to encourage research on vaccines against technologically distant targets, such as malaria; it can be usefully deployed as an incentive for individuals, groups, and organizations to solve the difficult biology problems implicit in the quest for a universal influenza vaccine. Establishing push and pull incentives would also drive private-sector engagement in demonstrating proof of concept and offset any potential concerns about the sustainability of the influenza vaccine market.

Successfully developing a universal influenza vaccine will require galvanizing intense and sustained effort across multiple partners toward a hugely ambitious goal, hence the committee's use of the expression "moonshot." This endeavor could be expanded to encompass a similar quest for a more broadly protective vaccine against coronaviruses with pandemic potential; that would be a substantial step toward reducing the societal disruption caused by pandemics and the current global inequities related to vaccine availability and distribution. Partnerships, such as CEPI, that involve governments and private, philanthropic, and civil society organizations could be incentivized to lead or coordinate the push for a universal influenza vaccine; for CEPI, an expanded mandate—accompanied by funding—would be needed for it to assume the leadership needed to create push mechanisms and foster pre-competitive scientific research.

Recommendation 5: The Global Health Threats Board or similar governance structure created by the G7/G20 pandemic preparedness and response agenda, working with other relevant organizations, should initiate a dedicated "moonshot" program to incentivize development,

licensure, and eventual procurement of a universal influenza vaccine candidate as a matter of priority. This program's structure and funding should include (1) a push element for universal influenza vaccine research and development, which could be led by a variety of entities, including the Coalition for Epidemic Preparedness Innovations with input from its Scientific Advisory Committee, the Biomedical Advanced Research and Development Authority, the HERA Incubator, the World Health Organization, the U.S. Centers for Disease Control and Prevention, or other agencies that operate beyond the vaccine exploratory science phase and have a stake in market shaping, and (2) a complementary pull element (an advance market commitment [AMC]) to ensure procurement of resultant universal influenza vaccines, with technical leadership from Gavi and the United Nations Children's Fund (as a procurement agency for Gavi). This influenza moonshot should be coupled with a parallel effort for coronaviruses or other respiratory viruses with pandemic potential that produce variants of concern. Financing for the push and pull elements for both virus families should

a. Receive funding from multilateral actors, development banks, philanthropies (e.g., the Wellcome Trust and the Bill & Melinda Gates Foundation), and regional governance structures, including but not limited to the Organisation for Economic Co-operation and Development, G20, World Bank/International Monetary Fund, regional development banks, the World Trade Organization, European Union, and African Union. This funding should be separately and individually supported by trade and global financing institutions of the United States, China, and the European Union, such as the European Investment Bank and Asian Infrastructure Investment Bank.
b. Include participation from middle-income countries (MICs). The price for participation for these countries should be value-based and tiered; it should be determined by a value assessment (e.g., Health Technology Assessment) as part of the AMC. A financial intermediary such as a multilateral development bank should underwrite MICs' own value-based AMCs, so countries do not need to put aside scarce resources until an effective product is approved.
c. Include country-specific tiered prices for guaranteed volumes of vaccines to multiple developers that meet the minimum efficacy threshold, to provide an incentive to retain multiple potential innovators. This would hedge risk against late failure of one or more early candidates and protect against the possibility of safety risks after widespread deployments that require restricted use or result in the first entrant's withdrawal from the market.

d. **Include a requirement for successful vaccine innovator(s) to license their vaccines to other suppliers or manufacturers at low or zero cost, as a condition of accessing this guaranteed market. This will help facilitate widespread scale-up across all countries.**
e. **Be carefully costed over the next 1–2 years, to determine the scale of funding for this moonshot that could reasonably derisk investments in influenza vaccine technologies.**

Manufacturing Scale-Up and Supporting Geographically Distributed Hubs for Influenza Vaccine Manufacturing and Supply Chain Capacity

Regional or "geographically distributed" manufacturing hubs offer promise in helping counter vaccine nationalism and promoting equitable access through self-sufficiency. However, distributing manufacturing does not offer a full solution for addressing issues of vaccine equity, and it should be balanced with increasing the overall scale of global vaccine production capacity that can be applied to producing pandemic vaccines. Greater scale in global manufacturing capacity reduces the probability and likely extent of rationing in a pandemic; greater geographic distribution of that capacity reduces the inequalities of access that might arise from such rationing. Moreover, vaccine manufacturing capacity is not entirely fungible. As it is difficult to predict the optimal platform for each pathogen with pandemic potential, it is also important to strive for diversification of the number of facilities, their locations, and the types of platforms they can manufacture.

Distributed manufacturing hubs face several barriers to sustainability and success: they (1) require strong government commitment and industry involvement, (2) must comply with Good Manufacturing Practices and operate in a robust policy and regulatory environment, (3) require a strong business model (in terms of both demand for vaccines *and* the potential to manufacture other products for regional or global needs or keep production of pandemic or other vaccines at levels high enough for the facilities to stay "warm"), (4) must undertake workforce training for technology transfer and regulatory capacity, and (5) must have a business case that includes a provision for national plans (who will get vaccines, where, and how). No global institutional architecture exists to handle manufacturing coordination and market-based issues.

A business model for pandemic influenza vaccines requires a business plan for keeping manufacturing facilities functioning and sustained between pandemics. Current demands for seasonal influenza vaccine vary widely among countries and are not sufficient to support the expansion required to meet pandemic demands. However, if the technology platforms are appropriate for making vaccines for other pathogens, vaccines could be produced during times of no disease pandemics for other priority pathogens, such as Middle East respiratory syndrome, Zika, Ebola, and dengue, or current diseases that require routine immunization (e.g., polio). Physical factories and research facilities might also be used for products other than vaccines, such as mRNA-based therapeutics. Newly built factories and facilities will also need to have the flexibility to diversify their production, adopt a culture of Good Manufacturing Practices, and develop strong regulatory oversight. In addition to providing critical ingredients and manufacturing components, geographically distributed supply chain hubs present a market opportunity for countries to invest as suppliers of the bags, filters, and other items required for vaccine supply chains.

Recommendation 6: The Global Health Threats Board or similar governance structure created by the G7/G20 pandemic preparedness response agenda should initiate a *long-term* (10–20+ years) multilateral partnership to track emerging technologies that may be targets for technology transfer for vaccines for influenza; promote industry partnerships with geographically distributed hubs; and provide technical training. To do so, it should do the following:

a. **Identify or create an international entity to assume responsibility for catalyzing voluntary technology transfer initiatives for platform technologies, including influenza vaccines. The structure's governance should build on both the World Health Organization's and COVAX's work on the COVID-19 mRNA hub, expanding it to include a diverse portfolio of technologies capable of providing protection against diverse threats with pandemic potential, and the COVAX Vaccine Manufacturing Taskforce, expanding it to work with vaccine manufacturing bodies to identify supply chain inputs and needs across a variety of vaccine candidates.**
b. **Ensure that this entity promotes the development of platforms suited to the production of vaccines for other pathogens of national or regional importance in addition to seasonal influenza—or products such as therapeutics—including tracking technologies coming onto the market and building platforms for voluntary industry collaboration.**
c. **Develop or assist with the development of plans for geographically distributed hub training requirements, such as vaccine regulatory needs and vaccine product sourcing.**
d. **Encourage countries considering warming their manufacturing capacity for influenza vaccines and vaccines for other pathogens with pandemic potential to consider whether their focus**

should instead be on building new production capacity of key manufacturing inputs for vaccine manufacturing.

e. Be given dedicated funding to support these activities from the World Bank and regional development banks, in conjunction with the International Finance Corporation.

Last Mile to the Goal of Vaccination: Generating Influenza Vaccine Demand Through Globally Coordinated Deployment Activities

Vaccines do not save lives; *vaccination* saves lives. Many countries, particularly LMICs, lack adult vaccine deployment plans, systems, and experience, including for seasonal and pandemic influenza. Even in countries such as the United States, COVID-19 has demonstrated how vaccine availability and success at achieving high vaccination rates are different issues—and that both present serious challenges. Countries need to build and sustain vaccine deployment capability, especially for adolescents and adults. This is essential for both attaining public health benefits and "warming" and not "chilling" market support for vaccines and related programs.

Vaccine financing programs often focus more on procurement than on supporting the programmatic infrastructure essential to ensuring that vaccines are effectively used in the field. Deployment activities require proper technical guidance, operational plans and capacity, and *designated* financial resources for vaccination operations to proceed effectively. UNICEF and Gavi are well positioned to take the lead on global coordination for vaccine deployment, particularly in LMICs, while WHO can leverage its expertise in providing technical guidance on national pandemic and vaccination planning and country readiness assessments. Countries must take the lead on developing the operational capacities necessary for vaccination programs.

Recommendation 7: The United Nations Children's Fund, Gavi, and relevant national and regional organizations (including governments) should be given funding explicitly allocated for introducing and deploying next-generation seasonal influenza vaccines to underpin scaled-up manufacturing capacity. The World Health Organization regional offices should urgently work with countries to do more extensive assessments of their readiness to reach appropriate populations, including adults and high-risk groups, to enable work plans by 2023, which include the following:

a. An analysis of what infrastructure (e.g., data and digitization of immunization records) built for COVID can be adapted, strengthened, and sustained for at least one additional adult and one adolescent vaccine.

b. **Advising member states on best practices used in countries that had high immunization rates during COVID-19.**
c. **Assisting member states to look at their data and logistics systems for monitoring coverage and for tracking safety (pharmacovigilance) and on the options for adopting no-fault compensation as part of patient safety mechanisms.**

Influenza presents a major pandemic threat, requiring urgent global coordination and partnerships. For optimal effectiveness, efficiency, sustainability, and impact, "countering the pandemic threat of *influenza*" should be reframed to "countering the pandemic threat of *influenza within a wider respiratory pathogen*" PPR framework. This move toward an integrated framework for respiratory pathogens with pandemic potential can only occur with large, dedicated financial investments, particularly targeting LMICs. Countering influenza is a global imperative on public health, economic, and equity levels.

REFERENCES

Anand, A., J. Sandefur, and A. Subramanian. 2021. *Three new estimates of India's all-cause excess mortality during the COVID-19 pandemic.* https://www.cgdev.org/publication/three-new-estimates-indias-all-cause-excess-mortality-during-covid-19-pandemic (accessed December 16, 2021).

BMGF (Bill & Melinda Gates Foundation). 2021. Global grand challenges. *Ending the pandemic threat: A grand challenge for universal influenza vaccine development.* https://gcgh.grandchallenges.org/challenge/ending-pandemic-threat-grand-challenge-universal-influenza-vaccine-development (accessed October 21, 2021).

Ewing, E. T. 2021. *Health Affairs Blog.* https://www.healthaffairs.org/do/10.1377/hblog20210329.51293/full (accessed July 16, 2021).

GPMB (Global Preparedness Monitoring Board). 2019. *A world at risk.* Geneva, Switzerland: World Health Organization. https://www.gpmb.org/annual-reports/annual-report-2019 (accessed December 16, 2021).

IFPMA (International Federation of Pharmaceutical Manufacturers & Associations). 2021. *Towards vaccinating the world: Landscape of current COVID-19 supply chain and manufacturing capacity, potential challenges, initial responses, and possible "solution space"—a Discussion Document.* https://www.ifpma.org/wp-content/uploads/2021/03/Summit_Landscape_Discussion_Document.pdf (accessed December 16, 2021).

Kelland, K. 2019. *World must prepare for inevitable next flu pandemic, WHO says.* https://www.reuters.com/article/us-health-flu-who/world-must-prepare-for-inevitable-next-flu-pandemic-who-says-idUSKBN1QS1EP (accessed August 19, 2021).

Kremer, M., and R. Glennerster. 2004. *Strong medicine: Creating incentives for pharmaceutical research on neglected diseases.* Princeton, NJ: Princeton University Press.

Lurie, N., G. T. Keusch, and V. J. Dzau. 2021. Urgent lessons from COVID 19: Why the world needs a standing, coordinated system and sustainable financing for global research and development. *The Lancet* 397(10280):1229–1236.

Palache, A., T. Tsai, Y. Vasiliev, A. Abelin, R. Hollingsworth, B. Taylor, and P. Barbosa. 2020. Global influenza vaccine distribution survey demonstrates urgency of implementation of Objective 3 of WHO influenza strategy 2019–2030. *Internal Medicine Review* 6(2):1–27.

Sparrow, E., J. G. Wood, C. Chadwick, A. T. Newall, S. Torvaldsen, A. Moen, and G. Torelli. 2021. Global production capacity of seasonal and pandemic influenza vaccines in 2019. *Vaccine* 39(3):512–520.

Taubenberger, J.K., and D. M. Morens. 2006. 1918 Influenza: the mother of all pandemics. *Emerging Infectious Diseases* 12(1):15–22.

Yeyati, E. L., and F. Filippini. 2021. *Social and economic impact of COVID-19*. Brookings Global Working Paper #158. Global Economy and Development program at Brookings. https://www.brookings.edu/wp-content/uploads/2021/06/Social-and-economic-impact-COVID.pdf (accessed December 16, 2021).

WHO (World Health Organization). 2019a. *Global influenza strategy 2019–2030*. Geneva, Switzerland: World Health Organization. https://apps.who.int/iris/bitstream/handle/10665/311184/9789241515320-eng.pdf (accessed October 21, 2021).

WHO. 2019b. *The public health implications of implementation of the Nagoya Protocol: Report by the Director-General*. https://apps.who.int/gb/ebwha/pdf_files/EB148/B148_21-en.pdf (accessed December 16, 2021).

1

Introduction: The Imperative for Global Investment in Influenza Vaccines

The year 2020 will be remembered as "the year of COVID-19" (Lurie et al., 2021). As of July 2021, the number of reported COVID-19 cases surpassed 184 million, resulting in more than 4 million reported deaths worldwide (CRS, 2021). The pandemic has created an economic crisis, which some scholars estimate may cost the global economy more than $10 trillion (Glassman and Smitham, 2021). Unemployment levels are currently comparable to the Great Depression of the 1930s, 95 million people worldwide are estimated to have entered extreme poverty in 2020, and an estimated 80 million more are undernourished relative to pre-pandemic levels. The global economic downturn has produced estimates of a 5.3 percent drop in global trade for 2020, imposing a particularly heavy toll on trade-dependent developing and emerging economies (CRS, 2021).

While scientists and public health policy makers may not have been able to predict that it would be specifically *SARS-CoV-2,* the cause of COVID-19, that would cause the next major pandemic, they *did* underscore the vital importance of preparing for a major respiratory pandemic due to an as-yet-unknown pathogen, or "Disease X" (Simpson et al., 2020). In its 2019 Strategy document, the World Health Organization (WHO) stated, "Although it is impossible to predict when the next pandemic might occur, its occurrence is considered inevitable, and it could well occur during the time frame of this strategy. Given increased economic globalization, urbanization and mobility, the next pandemic will spread further and faster, and could lead to significant disruptions" (WHO, 2019). That same year, the Global Preparedness Monitoring Board (GPMB) discussed "preparing for the worst: a rapidly spreading, lethal respiratory pathogen pandemic ... such as an especially deadly strain of influenza" (GPMB, 2019).

Despite the devastation wrought by COVID-19, from an epidemiological perspective, it does not represent a "worst-case" scenario. Epidemiologists use the R_0 ("reproductive number") metric to indicate how contagious an infectious disease is;[1] the 1918–1919 pandemic influenza had an estimated R_0 of 2.0–3.0, which is close to the estimated initial R_0 for SARS-CoV-2 (2.5, or a range of 1.8–3.6) (Petersen et al., 2020). With a similar case fatality ratio (CFR, a measure of how lethal a disease is) so far for COVID-19, the 1918–1919 pandemic,[2] and new variants of highly pathogenic influenza viruses circling the globe annually, one could argue that pandemic influenza reflects an even more dire risk to global and economic health than SARS-CoV-2. Indeed, according to the U.S. Centers for Disease Control and Prevention (CDC) guidance on "categories of viral severity," the transmissibility and lethality of COVID-19 place it as a category three and two, respectively, with category five being the most severe (CDC, 2007). Experts worry that the risk for pandemic influenza may be even higher during the COVID-19 era due to an increased risk of overtaxed surveillance and testing systems and predict that another major flu pandemic is likely in the next 10–30 years (U.S. Senate, 2017).

The year 2020 also saw "unprecedented" innovation and scientific collaboration that produced new technologies, such messenger RNA (mRNA) vaccines, resulting in 3–4 times more COVID-19 vaccine doses projected to be available by the end of 2021 than what was possible for *all vaccines* in 2019 (IFPMA, 2021).[3] These vaccines were able to be developed in record speed at least in part because of fortunate viral attributes, decades-long investments in mRNA technology research, and pre-pandemic research on the spike protein, the major target for COVID-19 vaccines (Ball, 2020). However, the next pandemic pathogen could have an R_0 of not 1, 3, or 4, but 12–18, similar to measles, and a CFR not between 1 and 10 but in the range of 40–80 or higher, like the viruses that cause untreated Nipah (WHO, 2018), Marburg (WHO, 2021a), or Ebola (WHO, 2021b) disease. Vaccine production could be more complicated than for COVID-19 if this

---

[1] R_0 is generally reported as a numeric value or range whereby an outbreak is expected to continue if the R_0 value is >1 and is expected to end if the R_0 is <1 (Delamater et al., 2019).

[2] These numbers need to be interpreted with care; for instance, we may wish to substitute CFR with infection fatality rate (IFR), as well as ultimately measuring mortality by way of overall pandemic *excess mortality*; see, for example, Ritchie et al. (2021) and He et al. (2020).

[3] The announced cumulative supply target of COVID-19 vaccines is up to 14 billion doses by the end of 2021. This represents 3–4 times the pre-COVID-19 annual global demand for all vaccines (3.5–5.5 billion) (WHO, 2019).

hypothetical pathogen—like influenza viruses—has a high rate of mutation or mechanisms for evading human immune responses.

Although promising new technologies were advanced for COVID-19 vaccines, scholars have argued that collaboration across the research and development (R&D) ecosystem has largely "fumbled" during the pandemic (Lurie et al., 2021). For instance, the absence of global entities with a clear mandate, responsibility, or resources to initiate product development in a pandemic was exposed. No global organizations support a viral pathogen repository, host their sequence information, grow and share virus isolates for essential research, organize and collect biological reference materials from patients to support developing and validating new diagnostic tests, and incentivize manufacturing by buying raw materials. Some organizations, such as the Coalition for Epidemic Preparedness Innovations (CEPI), which was launched in 2017, have used their own resources to mobilize vaccine developers to pivot ongoing R&D to COVID-19. But they lack broad mandates to coordinate vaccine preparedness; CEPI, for example, could only fund early R&D and not late-stage trials. This has caused delays in vaccines reaching those who need them most and amplified distribution inequities. New multilateral frameworks, such as that of the COVAX Facility, have been launched to fill governance gaps, such as procuring vaccines for global allocation. These single-disease frameworks were largely reactive, lack permanent legal charters, and have faced issues with securing adequate financing from high-income countries.

In short, while experts knew in 2019 that a severe, novel respiratory pandemic could be on the horizon, pandemic preparedness governance writ large has been largely a "conductor-less orchestra." In Lurie's words, the COVID-19 pandemic has laid bare the "fragility of our global system of preparedness and response to pandemics, and the fragmentation of our research and development ecosystem" (Lurie et al., 2021). Economies across the world have been crippled by COVID-19, and yet it is far from the "worst-case" scenario for a future pandemic of "Disease X."

WHAT IF 2020 HAD BEEN THE "YEAR OF INFLUENZA" INSTEAD?

New strains of influenza emerge each year, but it is far from a new threat. This—and the fact that the influenza virus has a large animal reservoir and high mutation rate, making it difficult to predict which strains will circulate worldwide and decreasing average vaccine efficacy[4]—has

[4] Efficacy is the performance of an intervention under ideal and controlled circumstances (Singal et al., 2014).

often led to public complacency and intermittent buy-in for influenza pandemic preparedness efforts. Despite advances in vaccines and therapeutics, an estimated 1 billion cases of seasonal influenza annually occur worldwide (WHO, 2019). This amounts to a global incidence in almost an eighth of the world's population every year (Palache et al., 2020). Three to 5 million of these are severe and, on average, 290,000–650,000 lead to respiratory deaths (GBD 2017 Influenza Collaborators, 2019; Ruscio et al., 2020). Furthermore, these are likely underestimates because major gaps remain in data available to estimate the burden of influenza, particularly in low- and middle-income countries (LMICs) (Bresee et al., 2018; WHO, 2021c).

Pandemic strains of influenza are capable of high lethality; the 1918–1919 pandemic had an estimated death toll of up to 50 million (WHO, 2019). In the United States alone, if COVID-19 caused deaths at the same rate, the total death toll would approach 2 million (Ewing, 2021). Influenza pandemics occurred in 1957–1958, 1968–1969, and 2009–2010, resulting in 1–4 million, 1–4 million, and 100,000–400,000 deaths, respectively. Collectively, influenza pandemics can also cause consistently high economic burdens (see Table 1-1). The 2009 H1N1 pandemic, for instance, is estimated to have cost \$45–\$55 billion despite its comparatively low lethality. The World Bank has estimated that a global influenza pandemic with the scale and virulence of 1918 influenza would cost the modern world economy US\$3 trillion, or up to 4.8 percent of the global gross domestic product (GDP); even a moderately virulent pandemic would amount to a 2.2 percent loss of global GDP; and losses in sub-Saharan Africa would be equivalent to 1 year's worth of economic growth (GPMB, 2019).

In such a context, investing in pandemic preparedness—and particularly vaccination—is among the "best buys" in global health and the most cost-effective investment possible (Gouglas et al., 2018; The Rockefeller Foundation, 2021).[5] Yet, worldwide influenza vaccine[6] distribution before COVID-19 remained highly variable geographically (see Figure 1-1). This is both a demand and supply issue. Many countries, particularly LMICs, do not know the health and economic burden of seasonal influenza, have

[5] Considering the vast sums spent so far on domestic stimulus and pandemic suppression in developed countries—\$1.9 trillion in the most recent U.S. stimulus package alone—the sum needed for more comprehensive immunization is minimal, especially when weighed against the cost of another infection surge.

[6] Looking at seasonal vaccine access is an important proxy for pandemic influenza vaccines because it appears that COVID-19 may have increased acceptance of influenza vaccination in previously unvaccinated individuals and may have motivated uptake in newly eligible candidates. See Bachtinger et al. (2021).

TABLE 1-1 Snapshot of Estimated Economic Costs of Pandemics

Pandemic/ Epidemic	Financial Losses (US$)	Type of Calculation	Study	Citation
H1N1 (1918)	GDP losses: 3 percent (Australia), 15 percent (Canada), 17 percent (United Kingdom), 11 percent (United States)	productivity loss	McKibbin and Sidorenko (2006)	Yamey et al. (2017)
SARS (2003)	$52.2 billion*	productivity loss	Lee and McKibbin (2004)	Yamey et al. (2017)
H1N1 (2009)	$45,000,000–$55,000,000	total cost	Resolve to Save Lives (2019)	GPMB (2019)
Ebola (2013)	$2.8 billion (Guinea, Liberia, and Sierra Leone)	economic and social impact	World Bank 2014–2015 West Africa Ebola crisis: impact update	Yamey et al. (2017)
Ebola (2014–2016)	$53 billion	economic and social impact	Huber et al. (2018)	GPMB (2019)
Ebola (2014–2016)	$4.3 billion	lost productivity and trade	CDC (2019)	NASEM (2019)
COVID-19 (2020–2021)	$10.3 trillion (estimate)	forgone output	Glassman and Smitham (2021)	Glassman and Smitham (2021)
COVID-19 (2020–2021)	$11 trillion	forgone output	Georgieva (2020)	The Rockefeller Foundation (2021)
Expected cost: influenza pandemic akin to the scale and virulence of the 1918 pandemic	$3 trillion	not given	Frangoul (2014)	GPMB (2019)
Expected cost: influenza pandemic akin to the scale and virulence of the 1918 pandemic	$500 billion	intrinsic losses	Fan et al. (2018)	NASEM (2019)

* The calculations suggest that the cost in 2003 of SARS for the world economy as a whole is close to $US40 billion.

national influenza vaccination plans and programs, especially for adults, or prioritized seasonal influenza vaccination. For example, in 2009, the estimate of worldwide capacity for producing monovalent[7] pandemic influenza vaccines was 2.7 billion doses compared to the total worldwide population of approximately 6.85 billion, enough doses for approximately one-third of that population. By 2019, this capacity had risen to approximately 6.4 billion doses, or enough to inoculate about three-quarters of the global population, in large part due to the efforts of WHO's Global Action Plan for Influenza Vaccines (GAP, see Chapter 2) and improved vaccine technologies, such as increasing the use of adjuvants (Rockman et al., 2020).

What would the global community have done to scale up influenza vaccine production if we were experiencing a pandemic influenza strain with relatively high lethality (1–2 percent) this year? Chapter 3 includes more detail about where influenza vaccine manufacturing partnerships are taking place and how they have evolved over the past 15 years. As of 2019, approximately 79 percent of pandemic influenza vaccine production capacity (and 80–95 percent of seasonal influenza vaccine production) uses egg-based systems, which means that pandemic influenza vaccine production takes time; the large caveat for the above estimate that 6.4 billion

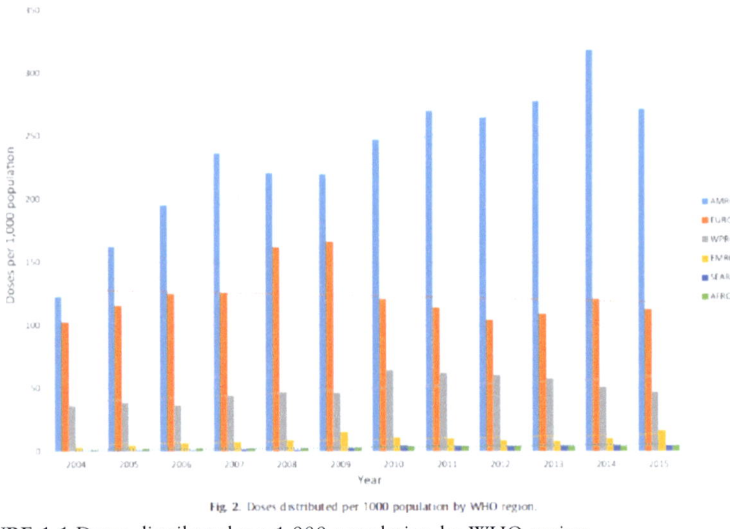

FIGURE 1-1 Doses distributed per 1,000 population by WHO region.
SOURCE: Palache et al., 2021 (CC BY-NC-ND 4.0).

[7] Monovalent vaccines contain a single strain of a single antigen; polyvalent vaccines contain two or more strains/serotypes of the same antigen (WHO, 2021d).

influenza vaccines[8] could be produced during a pandemic is that it is based on a full year's manufacturing output. Realistically, it would take about 3–6 months for full-scale manufacturing to begin, because it requires preparing and testing a suitable viral strain, and another 6–9 months to scale up to full capacity. Modern vaccine platform technologies, such as recombinant proteins and mRNA, can produce more quickly than egg-based systems and may improve yields because they do not require the full pandemic virus or candidate vaccine virus and are not limited by the supply of embryonated eggs available to grow viral strains. Since 2009, the number of manufacturers has also increased (as of 2020, at least 32 had licensed influenza vaccines), but a full two-thirds of the total was still produced by only seven manufacturers, most of them in wealthy countries (Rockman et al., 2020; Sparrow et al., 2021).

If it had been a new pandemic influenza virus that circulated this year, the potential vaccine production capacity could, therefore, have been available in a high enough volume to cover most vulnerable populations worldwide. However, this is largely theoretical; it assumes that surveillance systems would quickly identify the spillover virus, the country in which the virus was identified would be willing to share viral samples or sequence information, the pandemic strain would grow as well in eggs or cell cultures as seasonal influenza strains, and a clear—and early—signal would appear for manufacturers to switch from producing seasonal to pandemic influenza vaccines. (That ability to switch could also be affected by how far seasonal vaccine production has progressed; it diminishes as seasonal production advances.) It also assumes that the pandemic virus would supplant circulating seasonal influenza viruses (so no need for seasonal influenza vaccines), that manufacturers would be willing to switch production, with the understanding that the market for seasonal influenza vaccines already in production would cease but a market for the pandemic vaccines would exist and that the vaccines would be affordable for LMICs. As of 2018, the WHO Pandemic Influenza Preparedness (PIP) Framework (see Chapter 2) had secured commitments from industrial partners to provide 400 million doses of vaccine for LMICs. This means that only about 400 million of the

---

[8] The most recent WHO analysis of pandemic influenza vaccine production capacity estimates it in terms of a "best-case scenario," 8.31 billion doses over 12 months, and a "moderate-case scenario," 4.15 billion doses on the same time line. The best case assumes manufacturers would operate at full scale with no limitations on supplies/reagents, pandemic strains would grow equally well in eggs and cell-based systems as seasonal strains do, and a moderate amount of antigen would be required to elicit an adequate immune response. The moderate scenario similarly assumes that manufacturers can all operate at full scale with no supply or reagent limitations and that pandemic strains would grow equally well; it departs from the best-case scenario by estimating that more (twice) the amount of antigen would be required than seasonal strains for an adequate immune response (Sparrow et al., 2021).

estimated 6.4 billion dose production capacity for the pandemic vaccines would have been explicitly allocated for low-cost distribution to LMIC member states through WHO, which is a drop in the ocean in terms of capacity needed (and these doses might only be delivered after the national needs of vaccine-producing countries have been met). Finally, it assumes that countries would have national influenza vaccination plans to direct distribution. As the most recent data show, these plans are highly variable across regions; in 2018, 85 percent of LMICs did not have national seasonal influenza vaccination policies or programs, which form the cornerstone for pandemic vaccination (Morales et al., 2021).

As David Fidler put it at the Readiness for Microbial Threats 2030: Exploring Lessons Learned Since the 1918 Influenza Pandemic workshop (NASEM, 2018), the global governance structures for influenza "may turn out to be gossamer strands across the mouth of a cannon." The world can produce more influenza vaccines today than in 2009 but has not yet solved the serious issues of vaccine access and equity and managing the "switch" from seasonal to pandemic vaccine production and the poor market-based incentives for producing influenza vaccines.

A DISRUPTIVE MOMENT TO RECONSIDER INFLUENZA IN THE WIDER PANDEMIC PREPAREDNESS LANDSCAPE

In many ways, the global health community entered the twenty-first century with optimism and a sense of shared will and values. As Farrar (2019) recounts, "There was clear political commitment to multilateral agencies, the United Nations, the World Health Organization and others as the essential international architecture that brought all the countries of the world together to share challenges and ensure, as far as possible, equitable solutions." But this era of biomedical achievements did not, in Farrar's words, serve "as the springboard to enhanced health for everyone everywhere, as science advanced with clear public and political support for ensuring the benefits of these advances in improving lives for all." The situation at the beginning of the beginning of the century's third decade is quite different. According to Farrar, "increasing nationalism and a retreat from a sense of common public good ... challenge the optimism of the first decade of the twenty-first century."

Some see the global health community as naively approaching pandemic preparedness with fuzzy notions about how acting for the public good alone will produce equitable access to vaccines and technologies. The reality is that good will and altruism are readily defeated by politics and money. Pandemic financing writ large has a poor track record in terms of sustained financing, which is often episodic and typically flows during a crisis and ebbs afterward (GPMB, 2019). During the 2014–2015 Ebola outbreak, for example, epidemic and pandemic preparedness increased to 16 percent of global health aid in 2015, then fell to 7 percent by 2017. Despite numerous new organizations, systems, and processes, particularly since the 2009 H1N1 pandemic, preparedness for an influenza pandemic and pandemics in general remains underfunded both nationally and through international funding mechanisms. In 2019, the Institute for Health Metrics and Evaluation estimated that it made up slightly less than 0.9 percent of development assistance for health (global health aid) (Glassman and Smitham, 2021).

The *Review on Antimicrobial Resistance* (AMR), established in 2014 by the UK Prime Minister and chaired by economist Lord Jim O'Neill, is perhaps the most poignant example of the challenges of attracting sustained financial investments for global public goods—even when they are considered high risk by epidemiologists and "best buys" by economists. The first AMR Review paper estimated that drug-resistant infections could cause the deaths of 10 million by 2050, at a total cost to the global economy of up to $100 trillion, and the final report called for urgent incentives for investment in antibiotics. Yet, a follow-up report in 2019 called progress "remarkably disappointing" and stated that "what is missing, despite endless words, is a firm commitment of monies from governments or pharmaceutical companies." As Chatham House summarized, the concern is that "governments are waiting for the crisis to escalate to justify large-scale spending on AMR, while pharmaceutical companies are waiting for governments to panic and start throwing more money at the problem" (Dall, 2019).

Could political will invigorated by the COVID-19 pandemic be harnessed to change this pattern and promote investments in influenza pandemic preparedness as a global public good? COVID-19 has produced a recognition of a need for strong incentive frameworks to balance the fact that sovereign leaders have the responsibility to protect their own country's populations first. Glaring shortfalls now on display during the COVID-19 pandemic appear to be triggering much-needed global action. For example, the U.S. Secretary of State, Antony Blinken, in remarks to the UN Security Council on February 17, 2021 (U.S. Department of State, 2021) announced an intent to "advance the creation of a long-overdue sustainable financing mechanism for health security, so we can leave the world more prepared for future outbreaks than it was for this pandemic." In remarks to the G7 in February 2021 (White House, 2021), U.S. President Biden announced actions to improve the health and safety of the U.S. population by protecting vulnerable populations worldwide. He called on the G7 partners to create a sustainable health security financing mechanism aimed at building the capacity to end the COVID-19 pandemic and prevent future ones. In addition, in January 2021, the G20 launched a High-Level Independent Panel (HLIP) on financing for global pandemic preparedness and response (PPR) (Italian Ministry of Economy and Finance, 2021). The charge to the G20 panel was to identify gaps in the existing financing systems for global pandemic prevention, surveillance, preparedness, and response and propose actionable solutions to address these gaps, leveraging resources from the public, private, and philanthropic sectors and international finance institutions. Although these measures are promising, their outcomes remain to be seen, particularly after the acute phase of the COVID-19 pandemic ends.

The enormous innovations in vaccine production that have emerged during the COVID-19 pandemic, including new technology platforms using mRNA and recombinant proteins, may hold the key to new vaccines for influenza—and for new markets to support sustainability for the many new vaccine manufacturing facilities created over the last decade. Yet, they may also lead to misguided optimism. Influenza viruses are biologically quite different from SARS-CoV-2, having much higher rates of mutation among other properties. Much R&D is required to establish the generalizability of the new approaches to vaccine manufacturing and to continue to develop the workforce necessary to sustain it. This approach will probably not be adequate in a world in which new pandemic threats can arise at any time with a potentially much higher R_0. On the other hand, care needs to be taken not to throw the baby out with the bathwater or consider the past too deeply. For all its defects and failures, the global influenza system is among the most well established and best functioning among the existing global health governance structures for infectious diseases (Carroll et al., 2021). Many elements of the system, which are reviewed in Chapter 2, are working as they were meant to and should be highlighted for this and possibly expanded to include other pathogens with pandemic potential.

Between March 2020 and May 2021, numerous efforts were mounted to understand the lessons of COVID-19 at the global, regional, national, and local levels. Many reports have been or will soon be issued to document these lessons and make recommendations for increased preparedness and effectiveness for dealing with future threats, including influenza.[9] These efforts are well grounded in science and robust analytics but tend to be focused on the past, including the COVID-19 pandemic over the past 18 months. The

[9] Such efforts include those by the U.S. National Academies of Sciences, Engineering, and Medicine (https://nam.edu/programs/advancing-pandemic-and-seasonal-influenza-vaccine-preparedness-and-response-a-global-initiative); the Lancet COVID-19 Commission (https://covid19commission.org); the IPPR Report by the University of California, San Francisco's Institute for Global Health Sciences: *The United States' Response to COVID-19: A Case Study of the First Year*, April 15, 2021 (https://globalhealthsciences.ucsf.edu/sites/globalhealthsciences.ucsf.edu/files/covid-us-case-study.pdf); the Pan European Pandemic Commission's Report *Rethinking Policy Priorities in the Light of Pandemics*, March 2021 (https://www.euro.who.int/__data/assets/pdf_file/0010/495856/Pan-European-Commission-Call-to-action-eng.pdf); and the G20 High Level Independent Panel on Financing the Global Commons for Pandemic Preparedness and Response (https://pandemic-financing.org/about-us). All websites accessed December 17, 2021.

current need is for recommendations that aim at countering *future* pandemics in ways that ensure significantly more effective measures than the world has been able to mount. It is easy to be reactive, but we need to be strategic.

Is this, therefore, a disruptive moment and an opportunity to truly rethink the whole system for managing respiratory viral diseases with pandemic potential? We may never have a better chance to undertake the required reforms. As the health, social, and economic consequences of a severe pandemic are now clear to all, the current push to increase and stabilize pandemic financing, partly inspired by COVID-19, may be either the latest rendition of the usual reactive pattern or the beginning of a genuine effort to achieve more effective governance and financing structures for sustained pandemic preparedness. The key may be to harness the current political will and momentum evident in the efforts of the G7, the G20, and many other groups to establish effective mechanisms for the longer term. However, this leaves open major questions. How should the speed of sharing viral samples versus equity in benefits (such as vaccine access) be handled? This is particularly salient due to recent policy proposals, such as the TRIPS intellectual property (IP) waiver and global pandemic treaty (Velásquez and Syam, 2021). What partnership models can help to keep platform-based technologies scaled up during COVID-19 "warm" (i.e., actively producing vaccines or other products) for influenza, and how can they be best coordinated globally? What scale of investment is required for pandemic influenza vaccination, and where should it be channeled? To what extent do the governance structures for influenza—often considered a "known" and non-dangerous disease—require reconceptualization if they are to attract such investments?

CHARGE TO THE COMMITTEE ON GLOBAL COORDINATION, PARTNERSHIPS, AND FINANCING

At the request of the U.S. Department of Health and Human Services, the National Academies of Sciences, Engineering, and Medicine (the National Academies) will spearhead an effort to assess the global impact that capabilities, technologies, processes, and policies developed for COVID-19 could have on pandemic and seasonal influenza global preparedness and response, especially regarding vaccine development. The content will be based on diverse evidence to ensure that the report can be contextualized, adapted, and implemented across various circumstances internationally. The effort includes four work streams that collectively will culminate in a comprehensive series of reports with recommendations to improve research and development, production, manufacturing, planning, scale-up, and timely distribution of influenza vaccines and countermeasures rapidly around the globe while protecting incentives for innovation.

To contribute to this effort, an ad hoc committee under the auspices of the National Academies will describe the current global governance landscape for influenza vaccines and vaccination; analyze the effectiveness and replicability of global coordination and financing models formed in response to recent viral pandemics and epidemics; and provide recommendations for governance frameworks, partnerships, and financing mechanisms that may promote sustainable influenza vaccine preparedness and response. Specifically, the committee will

1. Review existing global governance frameworks, partnerships, and intergovernmental treaties (e.g., the PIP Framework and International Health Regulations [IHR]) for seasonal and pandemic influenza vaccine development, manufacturing, and distribution, particularly those developed in response to H1N1, and identify any major barriers to the sustainable implementation of these frameworks and partnerships.
2. Review multilateral responses and public–private partnerships developed and implemented during COVID-19 (e.g., the ACT Accelerator) and other viral outbreak events (e.g., the Ebola epidemic), and highlight any approaches (e.g., R&D, liability frameworks, distribution, and innovative business models) that may confer significant advantages for national preparedness and regional and global coordination of seasonal and pandemic influenza vaccines and vaccination.
3. Drawing on the above reviews and the benefits and challenges presented by relevant global frameworks (e.g., the Nagoya Protocol and the PIP Framework), propose practical and feasible recommendations for sustainable governance frameworks and coordination mechanisms to increase global and regional preparedness for influenza; improve international influenza vaccine research, manufacturing, and equitable distribution and access; and address global challenges such as vaccine confidence.
4. Review the theoretical basis of incentivizing vaccine research, manufacturing, and distribution in the pandemic preparedness context, and identify any relevant examples of the successful and sustainable design and use of incentives, particularly for low-resource settings.
5. Provide recommendations for the contexts in which specific financing strategies and mechanisms (e.g., incentives, risk pooling, and trust funds) can be sustainably adapted. These mechanisms will ideally encourage national investment in pandemic influenza preparedness and response, while optimizing the effectiveness of development assistance for health.

The result of this study is a report on the current barriers to effective global coordination and sustainable financing for seasonal and pandemic influenza vaccines and vaccination and the ways in which innovations and lessons learned from the COVID-19, Ebola, and 2009 H1N1 responses may address these barriers. The Committee on International Coordination, Partnerships, and Financing will coordinate with other related initiatives, including the three other consensus study committees in this initiative, to ensure the widespread dissemination and monitoring of its recommendations.

To approach this broad—and time-sensitive—task, the committee held a series of meetings from March through July 2021. Four meetings focused on the existing major global governance frameworks and regulations related to influenza vaccination, gaps in and barriers to these frameworks and regulations, areas in which the committee could make recommendations to fill these gaps, and ways in which influenza governance and financing structures could be integrated with wider respiratory pathogen and pandemic governance infrastructures. A series of smaller meetings of working groups focused on pathogen sharing, global partnerships for technology and manufacturing, and vaccine financing and access. Each of the three working groups developed findings and conclusions in foundational areas to address the Statement of Task. Working group and full committee meeting sessions gathered information from 21 expert speakers, many with experience with responses to COVID-19, Ebola, and H1N1 influenza (see Appendix I for meeting agendas). The final committee meeting focused on revising crosscutting recommendations and delineating areas of paramount importance for future research that could not reasonably be addressed on the study's current short time line, such as vaccine confidence.

STRUCTURE OF THE REPORT

This report's recommendations are based on a single premise: starting with the first human detection of a novel influenza virus with pandemic potential, how can the global health community move as quickly as possible to develop vaccines and equitably immunize as many people as possible worldwide? This is not discounting the importance of the human–animal nexus; it was determined that analyzing such surveillance systems went beyond the reasonable scope and time allocation for this study. Chapter 2 provides a review of existing global structures, partnerships, and frameworks for influenza vaccination, including those that may detect viral spillovers from animals to humans. Chapter 3 also considers financing mechanisms that may improve surveillance in hot spot areas for spillover.

Four main steps were required to tackle this premise and make specific recommendations for improving influenza global coordination, partnerships, and financing mechanisms (see Figure 1-2). These steps correspond

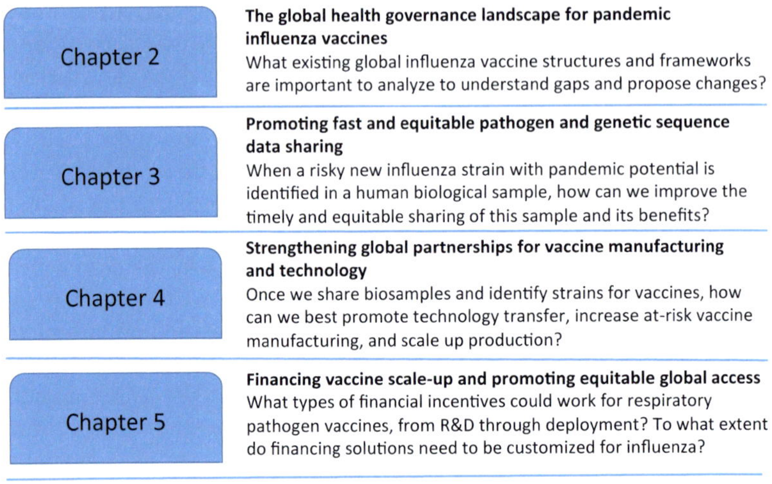

FIGURE 1-2 Chapter focuses and areas for recommendations.

to each of the upcoming chapters. Chapter 3 focuses on how, once a viral spillover from animals to humans is detected, the global community can ensure that samples are shared quickly but also as equitably as possible. Chapter 4 turns to global partnerships for vaccine technology and manufacturing; it considers, after pharmaceutical companies obtain relevant biosamples, what types of partnerships can best scale up manufacturing and create a sustained demand for vaccines. Chapter 5 focuses on how countries can ensure that the most people in the most places around the world receive vaccines as quickly as possible. It addresses the scale of financing and incentives required to improve access to influenza and other vaccines during a future pandemic. The concluding chapter presents the committee's recommendations and proposes ways to reframe preparedness for influenza pandemics to incentivize effective vaccine production and distribution in the post-COVID era and areas of the Statement of Task that should be prioritized by policy makers or further studied.

Across all chapters, the committee considers the areas in which the solution for pandemic influenza PPR should focus on influenza specifically and where influenza vaccination is best approached as a subset of solutions for broader respiratory pandemics. Ultimately, the committee argues that influenza presents a major pandemic threat and that addressing it will require enhanced global coordination, partnerships, and financing for respiratory pathogen PPR, particularly vaccines. Countering influenza is a global imperative for not only public health and economic reasons but also equity reasons.

REFERENCES

Bachtiger, P., A. Adamson, J. J. Chow, R. Sisodia, J. K. Quint, and N. S. Peters. 2021. The impact of the COVID-19 pandemic on the uptake of influenza vaccine: UK-wide observational study. *JMIR Public Health Surveillance* 7(4):e26734.

Ball, P. 2020. The lightning-fast quest for COVID vaccines—and what it means for other diseases. *Nature* 589:16–18.

Bresee, J., J. Fitzner, H. Campbell, C. Cohen, V. Cozza, J. Jara, A. Krishnan, and V. Lee. 2018. Progress and remaining gaps in estimating the global disease burden of influenza. *Emerging Infectious Diseases* 24(7):1173–1177.

Carroll, D., S. Morzaria, S. Briand, C. K. Johnson, D. Morens, K. Sumption, O. Tomori, and S. Wacharphaueasadee. 2021. Preventing the next pandemic: The power of a global viral surveillance network. *BMJ* 372:n485.

CDC (U.S. Centers for Disease Control and Prevention). 2007. *Interim pre-pandemic planning guidance: Community strategy for pandemic influenza migration in the United States—early, targeted, layered use of nonpharmaceutical interventions.* https://www.cdc.gov/flu/pandemic-resources/pdf/community_mitigation-sm.pdf?fbclid=IwAR1sMmehOSZ8hHRKEPJEP2hUbkXbNMlS4sGRqQ7s5iLWOpyfQDErd4Wg_SE (accessed June 29, 2021).

CDC. 2019. 2014–2016 *Ebola outbreak in West Africa.* https://www.cdc.gov/vhf/ebola/history/2014-2016-outbreak/index.html (accessed October 23, 2021).

CRS (U.S. Congressional Research Service). 2021. *Global economic effects of COVID-19.* Report R46270. Updated July 9, 2021. https://crsreports.congress.gov/product/pdf/R/R46270 (accessed July 16, 2021).

Dall, C. 2019. *UK report cites lack of progress on AMR review steps.* https://www.cidrap.umn.edu/news-perspective/2019/10/uk-report-cites-lack-progress-amr-review-steps (accessed July 1, 2021).

Delamater, P. L., E. J. Street, T. F. Leslie, Y. T. Yang, and K. H. Jacobsen. 2019. Complexity of the basic reproduction number (R_0). *Emerging Infectious Diseases* 25(1):1–4.

Ewing, E. T. 2021. *Measuring mortality in the pandemics of 1918–19 and 2020–21.* Health Affairs Blog. https://www.healthaffairs.org/do/10.1377/hblog20210329.51293/full (accessed July 16, 2021).

Fan, V. Y., D. T. Jamison, and H. Summers. 2018. Pandemic risk: How large are the expected losses? *Bulletin of the World Health Organization* 96(2):129–134. https://pubmed.ncbi.nlm.nih.gov/29403116 (accessed October 23, 2021).

Farrar, J. 2019. Science, innovation and society: What we need to prepare for the health challenges of the twenty-first century? *International Health* 11(5):317–320.

Frangoul, A. 2014. *Counting the costs of a global epidemic.* CNBC.com. https://www.cnbc.com/2014/02/05/counting-the-costs-of-a-global-epidemic.html (accessed October 23, 2021).

GBD (Global Burden of Disease) 2017 Influenza Collaborators. 2019. Mortality, morbidity, and hospitalisations due to influenza lower respiratory tract infections, 2017: An analysis for the Global Burden of Disease Study 2017. *The Lancet Respiratory Medicine* 7(1):69–89.

Georgieva, K. 2020. A New Bretton Woods Moment (speech at 2020 annual meeting, International Monetary Fund. https://www.imf.org/en/News/Articles/2020/10/15/sp101520-a-new-bretton-woods-moment (accessed October 23, 2021).

Glassman, A., and E. Smitham. 2021. *Financing for global health security and pandemic preparedness: Taking stock and what's next.* https://www.cgdev.org/blog/financing-global-health-security-and-pandemic-preparedness-taking-stock-whats-next (accessed June 16, 2021).

Gouglas, D., T. Thanh Le, K. Henderson, A. Kaloudis, T. Danielsen, N. C. Hammersland, J. M. Robinson, P. M. Heaton, and J.-A. Røttingen. 2018. Estimating the cost of vaccine development against epidemic infectious diseases: A cost minimisation study. *The Lancet Global Health* 6(12):e1386–e1396.

GPMB (Global Preparedness Monitoring Board). 2019. *A world at risk: Annual report on global preparedness for health emergencies.* Geneva, Switzerland: World Health Organization.

He, D., S. Zhao, Y. Li, P. Cao, D. Gao, Y. Lou, and L. Yang. 2020. Comparing COVID-19 and the 1918–19 influenza pandemics in the United Kingdom. *International Journal of Infectious Diseases* 98:67–70.

Huber, C., L. Finelli, and W. Stevens. 2018. The economic and social burden of the 2014 Ebola outbreak in West Africa. *Journal of Infectious Diseases* 218(Suppl 5):S698–S704. https://doi.org/10.1093/infdis/jiy213 (accessed October 23, 2021).

IFPMA (International Federation of Pharmaceutical Manufacturers & Associations). 2021. *Towards vaccinating the world: Landscape of current COVID-19 supply chain and manufacturing capacity, potential challenges, initial responses, and possible "solution space"—a Discussion Document.* https://www.ifpma.org/wp-content/uploads/2021/03/Summit_Landscape_Discussion_Document.pdf (accessed October 21, 2021).

Italian Ministry of Economy and Finance. 2021. *The G20 establishes a high-level independent panel on financing the global commons for pandemic preparedness and response.* https://www.mef.gov.it/en/inevidenza/The-G20-establishes-a-High-Level-Independent-Panel-on-financing-the-Global-Pandemic-Preparedness-and-Response-00001 (accessed October 21, 2021).

Lee, J. W., and W. J. McKibbin. 2004. Estimating the global economic costs of SARS. In *Learning from SARS: Preparing for the next disease outbreak: Workshop Summary.* Washington, DC: The National Academies Press.

Lurie, N., G. T. Keusch, and V. J. Dzau. 2021. Urgent lessons from COVID 19: Why the world needs a standing, coordinated system and sustainable financing for global research and development. *The Lancet* 397(10280):1229–1236.

McKibbin, W. J., and A. A. Sidorenko. 2006. *Global macroeconomic consequences of pandemic influenza.* Centre for Applied Macroeconomic Analysis, Crawford School of Public Policy, Australian National University. https://cama.crawford.anu.edu.au/pdf/working-papers/2006/262006.pdf (accessed October 21, 2021).

Morales, K. F., D. W. Brown, L. Dumolard, C. Steulet, A. Vilajeliu, A. M. Ropero Alvarez, A. Moen, M. Friede, and P. Lambach. 2021. Seasonal influenza vaccination policies in the 194 WHO member states: The evolution of global influenza pandemic preparedness and the challenge of sustaining equitable vaccine access. *Vaccine X* 8:100097.

NASEM (National Academies of Sciences, Engineering, and Medicine). 2019. *Readiness for microbial threats 2030: Exploring lessons learned since the 1918 influenza pandemic: Proceedings of a workshop.* Washington, DC: The National Academies Press.

Palache, A, T. Tsai, Y. Vasiliev, A. Abelin, R. Hollingsworth, B. Taylor, and P. Barbosa. 2020. Global influenza vaccine distribution survey demonstrates urgency of implementation of objective 3 of WHO influenza strategy 2019–2030. *Internal Medicine Review* 6(2):1–27.

Palache, A., S. Rockman, B. Taylor, M. Akcay, J. K. Billington, P. Barbosa, IFPMA Influenza Vaccine Supply task force. 2021. Vaccine complacency and dose distribution inequities limit the benefits of seasonal influenza vaccination, despite a positive trend in use. *Vaccine* 39(41):6081–6087.

Petersen, E. M., U. Koopmans, D. H. Go, N. Hamer, F. Petrosillo, M. Castelli, M. Storgaard, S. Al Khalili, and L. Simonsen. 2020. Comparing SARS-CoV-2 with SARS-CoV and influenza pandemics. *The Lancet Infectious Diseases* 20(9):e238–e244.

Resolve to Save Lives. 2019. *A disease threat anywhere is a disease threat everywhere.* https://resolvetosavelives.org/assets/Resources/RTSL_Fact_Sheet_3_22_19.pdf (accessed November 4, 2021).

Ritchie, H., E. Ortiz-Ospina, D. Beltekian, E. Mathieu, J. Hasell, B. Macdonald, C. Giattino, C. Appel, L. Rodés-Guirao, and M. Roser. 2021. *Mortality risk of COVID-19.* https://ourworldindata.org/mortality-risk-covid (accessed April 18, 2021).

The Rockefeller Foundation. 2021. *One for all: An action plan for financing global vaccination and sustainable growth.* New York: The Rockefeller Foundation.

Rockman, S., K. Laurie, and I. Barr. 2020. Pandemic influenza vaccines: What did we learn from the 2009 pandemic and are we better prepared now? *Vaccines* 8(2):211.

Ruscio, B., A. Bolster, J. Bresee, and London Shaping Meeting Participants. 2020. Shaping meeting to explore the value of a coordinated work plan for epidemic and pandemic influenza vaccine preparedness. *Vaccine* 38(16):3179–3183.

Simpson, S., M. C. Kaufmann, V. Glozman, and A. Chakrabarti. 2020. Disease X: Accelerating the development of medical countermeasures for the next pandemic. *The Lancet Infectious Diseases* 20(5):e108–e115.

Singal, A. G., P. D. R. Higgins, and A. K. Waljee. 2014. A primer on effectiveness and efficacy trials. *Clinical and Translational Gastroenterology* 5(1):e45.

Sparrow, E., J. G. Wood, C. Chadwick, A. T. Newall, S. Torvaldsen, A. Moen, and G. Torelli. 2021. Global production capacity of seasonal and pandemic influenza vaccines in 2019. *Vaccine* 39(3):512–520.

U.S. Department of State. 2021. *Secretary Antony J. Blinken remarks to the UN Security Council briefing on COVID-19 and vaccine access.* https://www.state.gov/secretary-antony-j-blinken-remarks-to-the-un-security-council-briefing-on-covid-19-and-vaccine-access (accessed December 17, 2021).

U.S. Senate, Committee on Foreign Relations, Subcommittee on Multilateral International Development, Multilateral Institutions, and International Economic, Energy, and Environmental Policy. 2017. *Testimony of Dr. Rebecca Katz: The World Health Organization and Pandemic Preparedness.* June 20, 2017. Washington, DC.

Velásquez, G., and N. Syam. 2021. *A new WHO international treaty on pandemic preparedness and response: Can it address the needs of the global south?* Geneva, Switzerland: South Centre.

White House. 2021. *Fact sheet: President Biden to take action on global health through support of COVAX and calling for health security financing.* https://www.whitehouse.gov/briefing-room/statements-releases/2021/02/18/fact-sheet-president-biden-to-take-action-on-global-health-through-support-of-covax-and-calling-for-health-security-financing (accessed July 16, 2021).

WHO (World Health Organization). 2018. *Nipah virus fact sheet.* https://www.who.int/news-room/fact-sheets/detail/nipah-virus (accessed July 1, 2021).

WHO. 2019. *Global influenza strategy 2019–2030.* Geneva, Switzerland: World Health Organization.

WHO. 2021a. *Fact sheet: Marburg virus disease.* https://www.who.int/news-room/fact-sheets/detail/marburg-virus-disease (accessed July 1, 2021).

WHO. 2021b. *Ebola virus disease fact sheet.* https://www.who.int/en/news-room/fact-sheets/detail/ebola-virus-disease (accessed July 1, 2021).

WHO. 2021c. *Global influenza surveillance and response system (GISRS).* https://www.who.int/initiatives/global-influenza-surveillance-and-response-system (accessed July 1, 2021).

WHO. 2021d. *Vaccine safety basics.* https://vaccine-safety-training.org/types-of-vaccine.html (accessed December 17, 2021).

Yamey, G., M. Schaferhoff, O. K. Aars, B. Bloom, D. Carroll, M. Chawla, V. Dzau, R. Echalar, I. S. Gill, T. Godal, S. Gupta, D. Jamnison, P. Kelley, F. Kristenen, C. Mundaca- Shah, B. Oppenheim, J. Pavlin, R. Salvado, P. Sands, R. Schmunis, A. Soucat, L. Summers, A. El Turabi, R. Waldman, and E. Whiting. 2017. Financing of international collective action for epidemic and pandemic preparedness. *The Lancet Global Health* 5(8):E742–E744. https://www.thelancet.com/journals/langlo/article/PIIS2214-109X(17)30203-6/fulltext#articleInformation (accessed October 23, 2021).

2

The Existing Global Governance Landscape for Influenza Vaccines

WORLD HEALTH ORGANIZATION AND THE INFLUENZA "REGIME COMPLEX"

Global health governance structures and frameworks for pandemic preparedness have often been developed reactively. In recent years, major outbreaks and pandemics have resulted in new international agreements and reforms; the International Health Regulations (IHR) revisions were rolled out in 2005 in response to the severe acute respiratory syndrome (SARS) outbreak of 2002–2003, the 2009 H1N1 pandemic led to discussions that ultimately resulted in a new access and benefit sharing (ABS) system for influenza, and the World Health Organization (WHO) research and development (R&D) blueprint was a reaction to the 2013–2014 Ebola epidemic in West Africa. This reactive dynamic does not mean that pandemic preparedness and response (PPR) efforts have lacked strategic grounding, such as linking "health" to the less altruistic (and potentially more lucrative) goal of "security." However, such strategies were not sufficiently effective to attract the resources required to respond to the COVID-19 pandemic—and a window for "strategic reactivity" may now exist for pandemic preparedness and influenza governance. In David Fidler's words (NASEM, 2018), the global governance infrastructure for pandemic influenza may be best thought of as a "regime complex: a set of interlinked and overlapping institutions, rules, processes, and practices." It provides a web of PPR activities at both the functional and strategic levels. Governance mechanisms enable surveillance, virus sharing, scientific research, and vaccine development. Strategically, the "ecosystem" also integrates national security, economic interests, human rights, and ethics into pandemic influenza governance.

Much of the global infrastructure for pandemic preparedness is based on the scaffolds provided by long-standing governance structures for influenza. The first influenza vaccines were developed in 1942, and the newly minted WHO initiated the Global Influenza Program (GIP) in 1947. The Global Influenza Surveillance Network (GISN)—renamed the "Global Influenza Surveillance and Response System" (GISRS) in 2011—was launched under the auspices of GIP in 1952, with the recognition that more needed to be done globally to monitor changes in influenza viruses (Monto, 2017). As Hay and McCauley (2018) argue, the precise modus operandi of GISRS has changed over the years, but it has consistently been a mechanism for monitoring global influenza viral activity, identifying strains for annual vaccines, and forecasting potential pandemic threats.

GISRS is based on a largely "informal autonomous trust-based system" of laboratories and collaborating centers coordinated by WHO. The backbone of this network consists of approximately 143 National Influenza Centres (NICs) spread across 101 GISRS-participating countries that provide continuous surveillance of influenza. The NICs collect, analyze, and classify biological samples to monitor which strains are causing illness, how efficiently these strains are spreading, and how well previous vaccines have worked to combat their targeted viruses. Information is then disseminated through the FluNet database. These smaller centers pass the results from their wide-reaching investigations to one of six WHO Collaborating Centres (WHO CCs) for Reference and Research on Influenza, which provide more in-depth analysis of strains. GISRS then aggregates the data from FluNet and collaborators to predict the prevalence of influenza strains and allow WHO to select 3–4 strains to use in seasonal vaccines (Hay and McCauley, 2018; Ziegler et al., 2018). About 60 percent of countries now participate in WHO-mediated global influenza surveillance, supporting the IHR requirement for member states to notify WHO of all human infections with novel influenza viruses (WHO, 2008). GISRS is widely seen as one of the more successful global disease surveillance mechanisms and is now being leveraged for a pilot program for respiratory syncytial virus (Broor et al., 2020; Carroll et al., 2021).

GOVERNANCE GAPS EXPOSED IN THE 2009 H1N1 "SWINE FLU" PANDEMIC

From 1997 to 2007, a series of avian influenza outbreaks brought international attention to WHO and GISN/GISRS. First, an H5N1 strain with a high case fatality rate emerged in Hong Kong in 1997. Its reappearance in 2003–2004 and spread to other countries raised fear of a highly pathogenic avian influenza pandemic, compounded by the 2002 SARS coronavirus epidemic and the threat of zoonotic H7N7 influenza (Hay and McCauley, 2018). Avian influenza fears led to a frantic period of vaccine development and global preparations for pandemic influenza, during which issues of equitable access to vaccines and benefits from research on influenza viruses made some stakeholders question the legitimacy of GISN/GISRS, which reached a peak when Indonesia refused to share its H5N1 virus samples with WHO because it believed that it would not receive equitable access to the benefits derived from them (Fidler, 2010). The persistent H5N1 threat called for a wider appreciation of vaccine operations and benefits, as governments began to stockpile vaccines and antivirals, and led to "greater government scrutiny of the fairness of the global system" (Hay and McCauley, 2018).

In March and April 2009, a novel strain of H1N1 spread in Mexico and the United States (WHO, 2012). This ultimately led to the first influenza pandemic of the twenty-first century, which is estimated to have caused 151,000–575,000 deaths (Rockman et al., 2020). Early reports of H1N1 outbreaks activated information-sharing networks among the numerous WHO surveillance units, and the GISRS backbone responded well, in terms of assessing epidemiological information provided by the NICs and characterizing the virus' antigenic and genetic characteristics at the WHO CCs. The U.S. Centers for Disease Control and Prevention (CDC) officially reported the first cases of H1N1 to WHO on April 18, 2009. On April 29, 2009, WHO convened an emergency committee under the authority of the IHR to make recommendations on whether a pandemic should be declared (Kamradt-Scott et al., 2018). As the cases increased at more than 200 locations around the world, preparations for vaccine production and other responses began. A suitable candidate vaccine virus (CVV) was selected relatively quickly (Ampofo et al., 2012); by late spring, the seasonal vaccine production cycle was nearly at its end and manufacturers were able to begin preparations for dealing with H1N1 (WHO, 2012).

Although it obtained quick surveillance data for H1N1 influenza, WHO did not officially declare a global pandemic until June 11, 2009. Soon thereafter, it launched the WHO Pandemic Influenza A (H1N1) Vaccine Deployment Initiative, which it later deemed to be the "first coordinated global response to an influenza pandemic" (WHO, 2012). Under this initiative, WHO coordinated the support of governments, foundations, and manufacturers to facilitate access to pandemic influenza vaccines in low- and middle-income countries (LMICs). Eventually, millions of vaccine doses, syringes, safety boxes, and other items were donated, and substantial financial and logistical support was pledged.

Despite this novel deployment coordination structure, the H1N1 experience is generally considered to offer a cautionary tale for the challenges of upscaling production of global influenza vaccines and deploying them during a pandemic. Box 2-1 summarizes major gaps in terms of international

BOX 2-1
Vaccine Governance Gaps in the 2009 H1N1 (Avian Influenza) Pandemic

The surveillance mechanisms in place in 2009 did their part to quickly and successfully identify the H1N1 pandemic virus, but vaccine development and distribution did not go as well. In 2009, the estimated global influenza monovalent pandemic vaccine manufacturing capacity was 2.7 billion doses. The world population at the time was approximately 6.85 billion, which meant that only approximately one-third of the world population could be immunized—even under the best circumstances. WHO launched a deployment initiative after the pandemic began, the first adult pandemic vaccine procurement and distribution program of its kind, to improve equitable procurement and delivery of vaccines.

By the end of the pandemic, only 162 million doses of pandemic influenza vaccine had been produced, of which 90 million were used (Moyer, 2010). Most recipient countries did not receive donated vaccines until after the peak in November and December 2009, and some were still receiving the vaccine a full year after it was first made available. As a consequence, demand for vaccines was often lower than anticipated; in Africa, only 4 percent of the population received the vaccine, instead of the planned 6 percent. In spite of these issues, WHO leadership did lead to distribution of H1N1 pandemic influenza vaccines to 77 countries, many of which vaccinated large fractions of their highest-risk populations. In South and Southeast Asian countries, 95 percent of health care workers, 86 percent of pregnant women, and 73 percent of people with underlying health conditions received the vaccine.

Governance and policy issues that contributed to this pandemic outcome include the following:

- **Pathogen sharing:** No global framework existed for sharing benefits, including vaccines, resulting from viral samples shared with the GISRS network (Fidler, 2010).
- **Manufacturing:** Egg-based monovalent vaccines had poor efficacy and took months to produce. H1N1 did not grow as well as seasonal viruses in eggs, which led to lower vaccine yields per egg and delayed production (Hampton, 2011; Knox, 2009).

coordination for producing and distributing vaccines. Production was not triggered quickly because the switch from seasonal to pandemic vaccine production was poorly coordinated and did not occur until after many seasonal vaccines were already delivered. High-income countries (HICs),

- **Procurement:** No structure existed for procurement of pandemic vaccines for LMICs, so a structure was developed reactively by WHO.
  - *Access issues*—LMICs first received doses 3 months after they were available, largely because wealthier countries entered into early procurement contracts. For example, the Australian government made it clear to the Australian manufacturer CSL that it must fulfill the government's domestic needs before exporting to the United States. The United States pledged on September 17, 2009, to donate 10 percent of its vaccine purchases to WHO, but on October 28, the U.S. Secretary of Health and Human Services reneged on this promise until all at-risk Americans had access in response to vaccine shortages created by production problems (Fidler, 2010).
  - *Liability issues*—Manufacturers worried about assuming liability for a new vaccine and required purchasers to provide protection from liability claims. Governments that received donated vaccine ultimately agreed to indemnify manufacturers, donor governments, and WHO (i.e., to pay compensation that arose out of claims of injuries)—but these agreements took time and delayed deployment (Broor et al., 2020; Fidler, 2010).
  - *Regulatory issues*—Donations from companies across a variety of countries meant regulatory approval also took time. Manufacturer Novartis, for instance, prequalified three H1N1 vaccines, made in three countries. For each vaccine, the national regulatory authority of the country in which it was produced, WHO, and the national regulatory authority of the receiving country had to approve its distribution through WHO (Broor et al., 2020; Fidler, 2010).
- **Distribution:** Many countries lacked adult vaccination plans, which created confusion and delays in delivering vaccines.
  - Countries who received WHO-donated vaccine mostly had little to no experience with influenza vaccines; this created bottlenecks in terms of developing plans to use vaccines, applying to WHO for donations, and granting customs clearance.
  - Gavi and other international organizations are mostly designed for pediatric rollout, and most countries had immunization systems entirely focused on young children but not those adults most at risk for severe influenza, such as pregnant women, the elderly, and health care workers (Hampton, 2011).
- **Financing:** Pledges to the $56 million initiative fell short of projected expenses, and actual commitments fell short of these pledges (WHO, 2012).

including the United States, set up procurement contracts with manufacturers and began receiving vaccines as early as October 2009. But the majority of vaccines were mostly rolled out after the peak of the pandemic in the fall; by then, demand was low, many doses were wasted, and many low-income countries received less than planned. The egg-based vaccine also showed generally poor efficacy, which exacerbated issues with public confidence and markets.

Fidler (2010) offered a particularly biting analysis of equity during the 2009–2010 pandemic: "in terms of vaccines for 2009-H1N1, donations from manufacturers and developed countries were not the product of real negotiations, given that WHO and developing countries had little leverage to influence developed countries other than rhetoric about equity, justice, and solidarity." In the end, wealthy countries

> only agreed to make donations *after* (1) they learned, unexpectedly, that a one-dose regimen would immunize adults, which doubled the amount of vaccine available; and (2) data from the northern and southern hemispheres revealed that the 2009 H1N1 virus was behaving as a mild virus and not a killer strain, which reduced the threat the virus posed.

These countries ensured that they had sufficient vaccine to cover their populations when pledging donations, and some—including the United States—postponed donations when they were not politically expedient.

Apart from its role with vaccine production and distribution, WHO faced criticism over the timing of its declaration of a pandemic (a necessary step to initiate the "switch") and its decision to remove pandemic influenza guidance from its website. Three independent panels found no evidence that WHO had engaged in inappropriate conduct but also recommended significant changes for its responses to health emergencies (Cohen and Carter, 2010; Flynn, 2010; Kamradt-Scott et al., 2018; WHO, 2011).

EXPANDING AND ENHANCING INFLUENZA SURVEILLANCE SINCE 2009

The governance and financing challenges during the 2009 H1N1 pandemic stimulated negotiations that led to the launch of the Pandemic Influenza Preparedness (PIP) Framework in 2011. This framework is a formal, but nonbinding, agreement between WHO member states to improve PPR, with a focus on equity and benefit sharing. Under its governance, when countries share influenza viruses with pandemic potential (IVPP) with GISRS, they are entitled to access specific benefits, including timely access to vaccines, derived from these viruses in a pandemic. The PIP Framework agreement only covers IVPP strains. Pharmaceutical companies who use virus data from GISRS for products (such as vaccines or antivirals) provide in-kind donations or discounted product doses to WHO for deployment during a pandemic and also partner contributions, which are used to bolster capabilities for PPR (such as surveillance) for low-income countries participating in GISRS. Chapter 3 includes more details about areas of success and persisting gaps in the PIP Framework.

Governance structures such as the PIP Framework and the Nagoya Protocol on Access to Genetic Resources to the Fair and Equitable Sharing of Benefits Arising from Their Utilization of the Convention on Biological Diversity (discussed further in Chapter 3) have yet to be tested in an influenza pandemic. The world can now produce more vaccines than in 2009 but has not yet developed governance or coordination mechanisms to solve serious issues of vaccine access and equity, including the "switch," poor market-based incentives for producing pandemic vaccines, and deployment and delivery.

Like access and benefit sharing, governance structures for the surveillance and monitoring of zoonotic influenza have evolved significantly since 2009. In 2004, the OIE/FAO Joint Network of Expertise on Animal Influenza (OFFLU) was founded during the peak of the H5N1 (avian influenza) crisis. WHO joined forces with the World Organisation for Animal Health (OIE) and the Food and Agriculture Organization of the United Nations (FAO) in 2006, with the launch of the Global Early Warning System for Major Animal Diseases, including Zoonosis (GLEWS). This became an early One Health mechanism, linking together the three organizations for event-based disease surveillance. The 2009 H1N1 pandemic provided momentum for OFFLU, and in 2010, the three organizations published a Tripartite Concept Note on "Sharing responsibilities and coordinating global activities to address health risks at the animal-human-ecosystems interface" (FAO-OIE-WHO, 2010). They named avian influenza as a major priority for this alliance along with rabies and antimicrobial resistance (Dauphin, 2015; FAO-OIE-WHO, 2013). Through OFFLU, representatives of the veterinary and animal health sector have taken part in biannual WHO consultations on influenza virus surveillance data since 2011 that analyze surveillance data and provide recommendations on viral strains to use for influenza vaccines in the upcoming season. In this way, OFFLU participates in GISRS (routine influenza surveillance) and provides data collected from OIE/FAO Reference Centers and national animal health laboratories to WHO. Creating pre-pandemic CVVs for human vaccines relies heavily on this zoonotic virus data (Dauphin, 2015; Mackenzie et al., 2014).

In recent years, momentum has been building for extending the GISRS and GLEWS event-based surveillance or creating "GLEWS+" and "GISRS+." GLEWS+ is designed as a cross-sectoral mechanism for conducting joint risk assessments for influenza and other zoonotic pathogens (FAO-OIE-WHO, 2013). The GISRS+ proposal is currently in its infancy at WHO. In WHO discussions during June 2021, it was suggested as a mechanism to build on and expand GISRS surveillance capabilities based on capacities developed and gaps identified during COVID-19 (see Figure 2-1). GISRS+

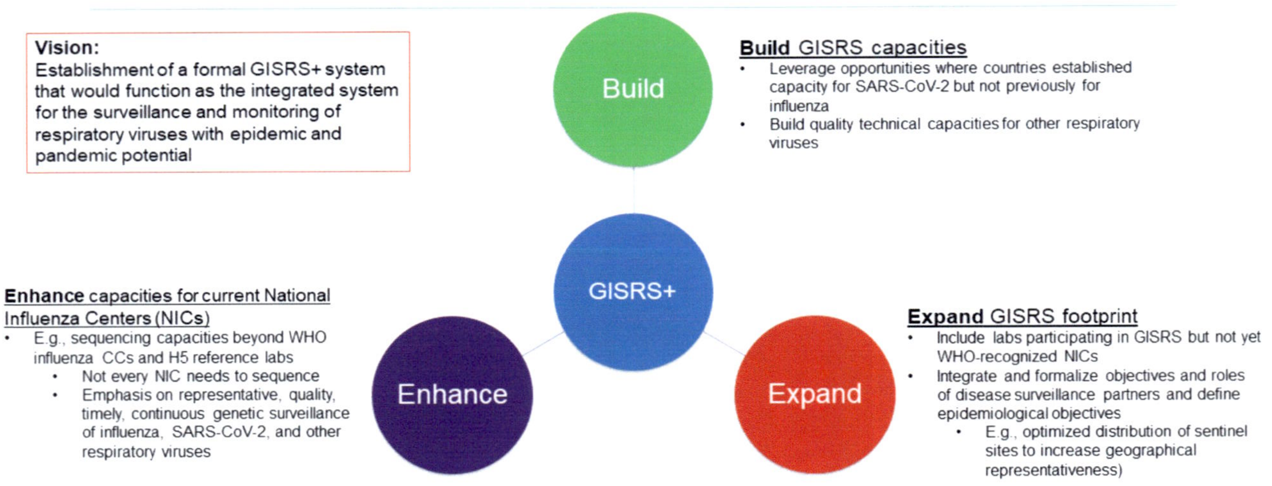

FIGURE 2-1 GISRS+ capacity building.
NOTE: CC = WHO Collaborating Centre; NIC = WHO National Influenza Centre; ORV = other respiratory virus.
SOURCES: Moen, 2021; WHO, 2021.

would function as the integrated system for surveillance and monitoring of respiratory viruses with epidemic and pandemic potential (WHO, 2021).

The GISRS+ proposal underscores the fact that GISRS structures have been leveraged during the COVID-19 response and can be expanded for other respiratory viruses. The laboratory network underpinning GISRS would expand, as would capacity building and training opportunities. Deciding which structures to extend (such as creating additional WHO CCs and how they will relate to GISRS) or redesign for other respiratory viruses (such as in the PIP Framework) will require a formal coordination mechanism. WHO is considering mechanisms required to support GISRS+ as a formal health governance structure.

A SNAPSHOT OF CURRENT INFLUENZA VACCINE GOVERNANCE STRUCTURES AND FRAMEWORKS

The WHO GISRS and PIP Framework form a major piece of the multilateral ecosystem for influenza surveillance and control. However, the wider "regime complex" or global ecosystem for influenza pandemic vaccines is much more complex and extends far beyond WHO's normative power. Box 2-2 provides a nonexhaustive overview of some of the major organizations and programs involved in global and regional influenza policy and governance (NASEM, 2018; Schroeder, 2018; WHO, 2019) based on whether they involve multilateral, bilateral, or regional coordination; international regulations; public–private partnerships (PPPs); industry partnerships; and civil society organization (CSO) partnerships. The structures highlighted demonstrate the often-blurred boundaries around seasonal and pandemic influenza vaccines and vaccination.

The list of organizations and programs in Box 2-1 reflects the 2019 Conference Report "Shaping meeting to explore the value of a coordinated work plan for epidemic and pandemic influenza vaccine preparedness," which called for a systematic effort to map the wide range of national, regional, and global actors that make up the influenza vaccine ecosystem (Ruscio et al., 2020). While this undertaking is beyond the scope of this short consensus study, it is an important next step. Our abridged analysis of major influenza governance structures reinforces that meeting's finding that strengthening influenza vaccine PPR must be "guided by an alliance of international stakeholders, to include, among others, governmental and nongovernmental organization representation, civil society representatives, vaccine manufacturers, international organizations, and health security and influenza experts" (Ruscio et al., 2020, p. 3179).

BOX 2-2
Major Influenza Policy and Governance Structures

Governance/coordination mechanism type

Examples	
Multilateral global	
WHO Global Action Plan (GAP) for Influenza	Phase I structures (2006–2011) had three objectives: increasing seasonal vaccine use, increasing vaccine production capacity, and expanding research and development. Phase II (2011–2016) focused on pandemic preparedness and technical objectives. The GAP Advisory Group recommended issues that required global coordination for vaccines and WHO leadership. Chapter 4 includes a case study of the GAP-mediated influenza technology transfer program for manufacturers.
Global Influenza Surveillance and Response System	GISRS is responsible for monitoring global influenza activity, forecasting pandemics, and identifying strains for the annual seasonal vaccine.
Global Vaccine Action Plan (2012–2020)	WHO, UNICEF, NIAID, and the Bill & Melinda Gates Foundation launched this plan to connect leaders across public and private sectors and increase equity in vaccine access. Influenza was only a small part of this plan, which—by 2017— had commitments from 197 countries' Ministries of Health. Most influenza work was focused on identifying gaps in research and policy (MacDonald et al., 2020).
OFFLU (est. 2004)	This is the World Organisation for Animal Health (OIE) and Food and Agriculture Organization of the United Nations (FAO) global network of expertise on animal influenza. It provides technical assistance and expertise to member countries to prevent, diagnose, surveil for, and control animal influenza. One main objective is to collaborate with WHO (through a tripartite agreement between WHO, OIE, and FAO) on issues related to the animal–human interface, including pandemic preparedness for the early preparation of human vaccines. WHO has been present as an observer on the OFFLU Steering Committee, and the OFFLU laboratory network is considerably smaller than GISRS (Dauphin, 2015).
Regional coordination programs	
Middle East, Eurasia and Africa Influenza Stakeholders Network (ME'NA-ISN, est. 2014)	This is a regional structure established to understand the current influenza burden in each member country and provide technical assistance with developing country–tailored action plans. Through meetings on National Action Plans, the network aims to strengthen surveillance, generate disease burden data, and help plan for influenza vaccine introduction.

Asia-Pacific Alliance for the Control of Influenza (est. 2011)	This is an alliance of Asian-Pacific countries, with an independent board of directors and members with regional expertise in influenza. Its objectives are to reduce the region's burden of influenza by addressing epidemiological issues and expanding local control initiatives, including vaccines.
International instruments	
Pandemic Influenza Preparedness (PIP) Framework (est. 2011)	This nonbinding framework brings together member states, industry, other stakeholders, and WHO to implement a global approach to influenza PPR. Its key goals include improving and strengthening the sharing of influenza viruses with human pandemic potential and increasing developing country access to vaccines and other pandemic-related measures. It was developed by WHO member states and unanimously adopted by the Sixty-Fourth World Health Assembly.
International Health Regulations (IHR 2005)	The IHR are a legal instrument binding all WHO member states that support the international community in the prevention of, control of, and response to acute public health threats, including infectious diseases. The revised IHR (2005) require countries to notify WHO about disease events that could constitute a public health emergency of international concern. They mandate reporting any case of human influenza of a new subtype B; require states to develop surveillance and response capacities; empower WHO to gather surveillance from nongovernmental authorities; authorize the WHO Director-General to declare a public health emergency of international concern and issue temporary recommendations; and seek to ensure the necessity of any public health measures that adversely affect trade, travel, and human rights.
Nagoya Protocol (est. 2009)	As an adjunct to the Convention on Biological Diversity, the Nagoya Protocol on Access to Genetic Resources and the Fair and Equitable Sharing of Benefits Arising from Their Utilization is an international agreement that aims at sharing the benefits arising from the use of genetic resources fairly and equitably.
Bilateral programs/partnerships	
National Institute of Allergy and Infectious Diseases (NIAID)	Part of the U.S. National Institutes of Health, NIAID works to "understand, treat, and prevent infectious, immunologic, and allergic diseases." NIAID has created the Collaborative Influenza Vaccine Innovation Centers network to coordinate and attract expertise to the effort to develop a universal influenza vaccine.
Biomedical Advanced Research and Development Authority (BARDA)	The National Strategy for Pandemic Influenza of 2005 designated the U.S. Department of Health and Human Services (HHS) as the lead agency for public health preparedness and medical response to a probable or actual influenza pandemic. BARDA, in the HHS Office of the Assistant Secretary for Preparedness and

continued

BOX 2-2 Continued

BARDA (continued)	Response, was established by the Pandemic and All-Hazards Preparedness Act in 2006 to facilitate the research, development, and acquisition of medical countermeasures for chemical, biological, radiological, and nuclear threats and emerging infectious diseases, such as pandemic influenza. As explored in Chapter 4, BARDA undertook major influenza vaccine manufacturing partnerships with WHO and PATH.
Global public–private partnerships (PPPs)	
Partnership for Influenza Vaccine Introduction (PIVI, est. 2013)	PIVI is a key program of the Task Force for Global Health. PIVI works in partnership with the U.S. CDC, Ministries of Health, corporate partners, and others to create sustainable, seasonal influenza vaccination programs in LMICs and with WHO programs to help countries prepare for pandemic influenza and support countries' efforts to control and prevent seasonal influenza (Bresee et al., 2019).
Global Initiative on Sharing All Influenza Data (GISAID, est. 2008)	This is a global PPP that provides open-access to the genomic data of influenza viruses and SARS-CoV-2, the virus responsible for COVID-19 (Shu and McCauley, 2017). GISAID was created as an alternative to the public domain sharing model, which traditionally does not offer protection of intellectual property rights to data or incentives for sharing (e.g., attribution of data owner). It is a platform for data sharing among WHO Collaborating Centers and NICs for the biannual influenza vaccine virus recommendations by GISRS. As of 2010, the Federal Republic of Germany is the official host of both GISAID and the EpiFlu databases (GISAID, 2020).
Coalition for Epidemic Preparedness Innovations (CEPI, est. 2017)	CEPI was launched at Davos as the result of a consensus that a coordinated international and intergovernmental plan was needed to develop and deploy new vaccines to prevent future epidemics. CEPI is a global partnership between public, private, philanthropic, and civil society organizations working to accelerate the development of vaccines against emerging infectious diseases and enable equitable access to these vaccines for affected populations during outbreaks. In March 2021, it announced a $US3.5 billion replenishment strategy and 5-year plan, aimed at cutting the vaccine production time line for new pandemics by two-thirds, to 100 days (CEPI, 2021). But CEPI has been more concerned with emerging pathogens, such as Chikungunya and COVID-19, than influenza.

Global Funders Consortium for Universal Influenza Vaccine Development	This consortium is a mechanism to bring together major funders of R&D for universal influenza vaccines along with key stakeholders to accelerate progress in the field through creating a common landscape, identifying critical gaps, and coordinating around a common vision. The consortium has created a database of novel vaccine candidates designed to provide broader and more durable immunity against circulating and pandemic influenza viruses and offer stakeholders and funders a common source of information to monitor research progress and identify opportunities for informed investments and collaboration.
Industry programs/partnerships	
International Federation of Pharmaceutical Manufacturers & Associations (IFPMA)	This global trade organization representing pharmaceutical industry members has an Influenza Vaccine Supply (IVS) task force, which is a specialized group of experts on influenza vaccine manufacturing. The largest manufacturers of influenza vaccines, Sanofi Pasteur, Novartis, Sequiris, ID Biomedical, and Glaxo SmithKline, are members and mostly based in the North American and European regions. The objective is to provide intergovernmental bodies and governments with expertise to guide pandemic and seasonal influenza vaccination; IVS has published studies of the global vaccine supply.
Developing Countries' Vaccine Manufacturing Network (DCVMN)	This is a voluntary public health–driven alliance of vaccine manufacturers from developing countries. Its goal is to improve the capacity of LMICs to produce vaccines and provide a consistent supply of high-quality vaccines for known and emerging infectious diseases that are accessible to these countries (especially public markets) (Pagliusi et al., 2020). DCVMN's vaccine contributions to Gavi markets increased substantially from 2012 to 2018, and, as of 2020, 15 licensed influenza vaccines were available from DCVMN members (Hayman and Pagliusi, 2020; Pagliusi et al., 2020).
Civil society programs	
Third World Network (TWN, est. 1984)	This independent nonprofit international research and advocacy organization is focused on strengthening cooperation among development and environmental groups, particularly in the Global South. Its work on influenza is centered on recommending policy changes to promote human rights, justice, and equitability. TWN was involved in PIP Framework negotiations and has taken active stances on influenza and COVID-19-related issues, including benefits sharing, bio-hubs, and intellectual property waivers.

THE GLOBAL INFLUENZA STRATEGY AND THE GOVERNANCE PATH FORWARD

Many efforts have been undertaken to distill lessons from the 2009 H1N1 pandemic for developing and rolling out vaccines, and there is, and will be, even more impetus to learn lessons from the COVID-19 pandemic. Given the centrality of WHO's role in coordinating pandemic responses, one of the most significant post-H1N1 developments was the WHO Global Influenza Strategy 2019–2030, which was issued in 2019 (WHO, 2019). In Annex 1 of the document, WHO discusses the achievements since the release of its first Strategy document in 2002. Annex 2 enumerates the areas wherein WHO sees ongoing challenges. The most relevant of these challenges, in terms of global vaccine PPR, are the following:

1. **Understanding influenza disease and economic burden:** Understanding the morbidity, mortality, and economic burden of influenza enables policy makers to prioritize influenza, make evidence-based decisions, and develop effective immunization and treatment programs. WHO states that most estimates of disease and economic impact have come from HICs, and additional studies in LMICs are needed.
2. **Undertaking consistent epidemiological and virological surveillance:** During the decade following the 2009 pandemic, GISRS was strengthened and improved. The number of member states sharing influenza viruses increased to 130 in 2017; member states sharing laboratory and epidemiological data through FluNet and FluID also increased. However, 31 percent and 58 percent of member states did not *routinely* share data on these respective platforms during 2016–2017. In addition, some countries still cannot detect novel influenza viruses, which is a core capacity under the IHR.
3. **Improving vaccine technologies and undertaking early and larger clinical trials that are more globally distributed:** Vaccines remain the most effective means of preventing infection and potentially reducing clinical severity. The reliance on embryonated eggs for production is still predominant, but, as described in Chapter 1, it is time intensive. Furthermore, some influenza viruses are increasingly unfit to grow and tend to undergo antigenic changes with passage in eggs, underscoring the need to diversify current production capabilities and technologies. The holy grail is a universal influenza vaccine that would offer broader protection against multiple influenza strains. However, as Fauci underscored in 2018 (NASEM, 2018), it will require long-term investments in advanced manufacturing techniques, such as cell-based production and new platform technologies. Pre-

pandemic clinical trials in adults and children may also inform the vaccination regimen required to induce a sufficient immune response for a novel influenza subtype, particularly next-generation viruses. This would reduce the response time for vaccine distribution if a similar subtype causes a future pandemic (Rockman et al., 2020).

4. **Building effective seasonal vaccination programs:** Because influenza viruses are highly prone to mutating, seasonal vaccines are strain based, and vaccination must be against the predominant circulating strains each year. WHO states that the need for annual vaccination, coupled with varying and often low vaccine efficacy, continues to contribute to influenza vaccine hesitancy. Both vaccine distribution and use also reflect major disparities. Recent data show that 47 percent of the global population (residents of countries in the Eastern Mediterranean, South-East Asian and African WHO regions) received only 5 percent of annually distributed vaccines. Countries and the global community must understand and address barriers that affect influenza vaccine distribution, uptake, import, and regulation to strengthen seasonal programs and improve the market for them if pandemic capacity is to be kept "warm" by seasonal vaccination.
5. **Performing national pandemic planning:** WHO developed pandemic influenza risk management guidance to encourage countries to develop national pandemic preparedness plans. In early 2018, WHO also published a checklist to help countries develop or update their plans. As of September 2018, however, few countries had updated their plans, and 101 countries did not have plans or had none publicly available. Without plans, countries would be hampered in terms of deploying vaccines during a pandemic (WHO, 2017).

In 2021, the Center for Infectious Disease Research and Policy (CIDRAP) took a step toward highlighting precisely how new technologies may be developed and harnessed for influenza. As discussed further in Chapter 4, its influenza vaccines R&D roadmap describes programs, policies, and financing that may accelerate progress for universal or broadly protective influenza vaccines. CIDRAP again underscores the importance of multi-sector and multi-actor collaboration for influenza governance; it is funded by the Wellcome Trust and advised by a steering group, composed of representatives of WHO, the Sabin Vaccine Institute, The Rockefeller Foundation, the Wellcome Trust, the Bill & Melinda Gates Foundation, and the Global Funders Consortium for Universal Influenza Vaccine Development (CIDRAP, 2021a).

The newest evolution of influenza governance may ultimately be through a pandemic treaty or instrument. The general concept of an international treaty on pandemic preparedness was put forward by the president of the European Commission in December 2020 and has been endorsed by the European Union, the WHO director-general, and 26 heads of state, although the United States has expressed a preference for a nonbinding agreement (Viñuales et al., 2021). In May 2021, the World Health Assembly reached a consensus to hold a special session in November, during which an international treaty or instrument on pandemic preparedness will be debated (CIDRAP, 2021b; Gostin et al., 2021). This proposal follows the general pattern of reactivity; it is a product of COVID-19 reflections that individual organizations and governments cannot adequately prepare for pandemic threats alone. This argument was taken up by the Independent Review Panel for Pandemic Preparedness and Response (IPPPR). In its May 2021 report, it recommended stronger leadership and better coordination for pandemic preparedness through a more independent WHO, creation of a Global Health Threats Council, and a pandemic treaty.

The pandemic treaty may best be viewed as a recognition that a future global health crisis response system needs to go beyond embracing the IHR and WHO as the global health coordination agency. Much work needs to be done on whether it would be modeled along the lines of the Paris Climate Change Treaty or the Geneva Conventions and what it would require under the auspices of a Global Health Threats Council and institutions such as the G20. More work will be required to determine its core functions and boundaries. For instance, some have argued that it should focus on "deep prevention" to reduce the risk of pathogen spillover from humans to animals (drawing on inspiration from the global governance of nuclear, environmental, and financing system risks) (Viñuales et al., 2021). Others have put forward concrete end points, such as establishing a global agency, similar to WHO, that can coordinate governments, launch large-scale operations, enforce international rules, assess health systems, and provide objective technical advice to countries (Moon and Kickbusch, 2021).

The pandemic treaty debate goes beyond the boundaries of this study on influenza governance. What we are interested in is how to best to ensure that the successful governance structures and frameworks used for influenza inform proposals being advanced by the plethora of groups and studies and that the specific requirements of pandemic influenza are given due weight as a highly hazardous pathogen. Our argument is that the global influenza system may well be the most well established and functioning among those extant systems for pandemic preparedness (e.g., GISRS for surveillance, the PIP Framework for ABS, GAP for vaccine manufacturing capacity building, and IFPMA IVS to provide a link to market generation). Some of these global arrangements and agreements can be made much more visible and prominent as examples that can either effectively withstand geopolitical tensions and sovereignty control or effectively operate sufficiently under the radar at R&D, technical, production, and trade levels.

Each of the next three chapters considers three interrelated questions. What is working for influenza vaccination, from a governance and financing perspective, and should stay specific to influenza? What is working for influenza and should be expanded or scaled up to improve integrated PPR for pathogens with pandemic potential? What is missing from the influenza vaccine governance landscape, and what partnerships or coordination structures could fill these gaps? Each chapter includes key findings and conclusions, which both respond to challenges laid out in the Global Influenza Strategy and form the basis for subsequent recommendations.

KEY FINDINGS AND CONCLUSIONS

- Global coordination for vaccines and vaccination will not be successful without including both public (national governments) and private actors—including civil society and the pharmaceutical and biotechnology industry.
- One of the key challenges for developing broader surveillance systems is how to cover multiple pathogens spanning the human and animal realms. Surveillance represents a prime example of how ministries and organizations, particularly those in the animal and health sectors, can develop misaligned objectives that contribute to silos based on the competition for influence, power, and funding.
- Programs supporting platform technology R&D and industry partnerships to scale up vaccines and address supply chain chokeholds are often performed in a semi-isolated context. This is true for influenza and other respiratory pathogens with pandemic potential. There is a need to move away from historically siloed systems toward a single architecture for the global coordination of PPR, in the spirit of the GISRS+ proposal.
- WHO and other international organizations cannot direct national ministries to take certain steps. They can, however, offer technical and managerial guidance, suggest policy solutions and mechanisms to facilitate multilateral agreements at the country level, and provide close follow-up.
- WHO is well placed to provide normative guidance, technical support for integrated surveillance, and regulatory support for vaccine licensure, for the coordination of global, regional, and national programs for PPR that recognize the importance of operating across multiple pandemic threats.
- WHO is less well positioned to support activities that require deep engagement with the private sector and industry, including vaccine manufacturing, supply chains, and deployment across multiple pathogens with pandemic potential.

REFERENCES

Ampofo, W. K., N. Baylor, S. Cobey, N. J. Cox, S. Daves, S. Edwards, N. Ferguson, G. Grohmann, A. Hay, J. Katz, K. Kullabutr, L. Lambert, R. Levandowski, A. C. Mishra, A. Monto, M. Siqueira, M. Tashiro, A. L. Waddell, N. Wairagkar, J. Wood, M. Zambon, and W. Zhang. 2012. Improving influenza vaccine virus selection: Report of a WHO informal consultation held at WHO headquarters, Geneva, Switzerland, 14–16 June 2010. *Influenza and Other Respiratory Viruses* 6(2):142–152, e141–e145.

Bresee, J. S., K. E. Lafond, M. McCarron, E. Azziz-Baumgartner, S. Y. Chu, M. Ebama, A. R. Hinman, A. Xeuatvongsa, S. Bino, D. Richardson, R. M. Porter, A. Moen, M. McKinlay, G. Sahakyan, S. Wangchuk, P. Ruowen, Z. Yongchao, C. Linlin, C. Daouda, O. Tarkhan-Mouravi, P. Gould, P. Muthoka, G. O. Emukule, S. S. Chaves, M.-A. Widdowson, D. Otorbaeva, V. Khanthamaly, K. Stavridis, V. Mikic, N. Furtuna, D. Capmari, B. Alexander, E. Dueger, M. Kamolzoda, J. Mott, A. Bin Salah, M. Mazur, A. Maria Ropero Alvarez, S. J. Olsen, S. Mirza, C. Sofia Arriola, J. Seward, S. Kluglein, A. F. Bolster, N. Minh Hang, J. W. McFarland, N. Ha Thu, and T. Thi Minh Nguyen. 2019. The partnership for influenza vaccine introduction (PIVI): Supporting influenza vaccine program development in low- and middle-income countries through public–private partnerships. *Vaccine* 37(35):5089–5095.

Broor, S., H. Campbell, S. Hirve, S. Hague, S. Jackson, A. Moen, H. Nair, R. Palekar, S. Rajatonirina, P. G. Smith, M. Venter, N. Wairagkar, M. Zambon, T. Ziegler, and W. Zhang. 2020. Leveraging the global influenza surveillance and response system for global respiratory syncytial virus surveillance-opportunities and challenges. *Influenza and Other Respiratory Viruses* 14(6):622–629.

Carroll, D., S. Morzaria, S. Briand, C. K. Johnson, D. Morens, K. Sumption, O. Tomori, and S. Wacharphaueasadee. 2021. Preventing the next pandemic: The power of a global viral surveillance network. *BMJ* 372:n485.

CEPI (Coalition for Epidemic Preparedness Innovations). 2021. *CEPI launches plan to tackle risk of future pandemics and epidemics*. March 10, 2021. https://cepi.net/news_cepi/cepi-launches-plan-to-tackle-risk-of-future-pandemics-and-epidemics (accessed July 7, 2021).

CIDRAP (Center for Infectious Disease Research and Policy). 2021a. *Influenza vaccines research and development (R&D) roadmap*. Minneapolis, MN: CIDRAP.

CIDRAP. 2021b. *WHA to hold pandemic treaty talks in November*. https://www.cidrap.umn.edu/news-perspective/2021/05/wha-hold-pandemic-treaty-talks-november (accessed October 21, 2021).

Cohen, D., and P. Carter. 2010. Conflicts of interest. WHO and the pandemic influenza "conspiracies." *BMJ* 340:c2912.

Dauphin, G. 2015. WHO/FAO/OIE tripartite coordination for the control and prevention of zoonotic influenza viruses: Example of OFFLU, global network of veterinary expertise. *Bulletin de l'Académie Vétérinaire de France* 168(3):224–232.

FAO-OIE-WHO (Food and Agriculture Organization of the United Nations-World Organisation for Animal Health-World Health Organization). 2010. *The FAO-OIE-WHO collaboration: Sharing responsibilities and coordinating global activities to address health risks at the animal-human-ecosystems interfaces. A tripartite concept note.* https://www.who.int/foodsafety/zoonoses/final_concept_note_Hanoi.pdf (accessed December 17, 2021).

FAO-OIE-WHO. 2013. *GLEWS+: The joint FAO-OIE-WHO global early warning system for health threats and emerging risks at the human–animal–ecosystems interface.* http://www.glews.net/?page_id=1041 (accessed December 17, 2021).

Fidler, D. P. 2010. Negotiating equitable access to influenza vaccines: Global health diplomacy and the controversies surrounding avian influenza H5N1 and pandemic influenza H1N1. *PLoS Medicine* 7(5):e1000247.

Flynn, P. 2010. *The handling of the H1N1 pandemic: More transparency needed.* https://assembly.coe.int/CommitteeDocs/2010/20100329_MemorandumPandemie_E.pdf (accessed October 21, 2021).

GISAID. 2020. *History.* https://www.gisaid.org/about-us/history (accessed October 23, 2021).

Gostin, L. O, S. F. Halabi, and K. A. Klock. 2021. An international agreement on pandemic prevention and preparedness. *JAMA* 326(13):1257–1258.

Hampton, L. 2011. *Why delivering COVID-19 vaccines might be just as hard as developing them: From liability laws to production delays, the 2009 H1N1 swine influenza vaccine rollout offers a cautionary tale for today.* https://www.gavi.org/vaccineswork/why-delivering-covid-19-vaccines-might-be-just-hard-developing-them (accessed July 6, 2021).

Hay, A. J., and J. W. McCauley. 2018. The WHO global influenza surveillance and response system (GISRS)—a future perspective. *Influenza and Other Respiratory Viruses* 12(5):551–557.

Hayman, B., and S. Pagliusi. 2020. Emerging vaccine manufacturers are innovating for the next decade. *Vaccine X* 5:100066.

IPPPR (Independent Review Panel for Pandemic Preparedness and Response). 2021. *COVID-19: Make it the last pandemic.* https://theindependentpanel.org/wp-content/uploads/2021/05/COVID-19-Make-it-the-Last-Pandemic_final.pdf (accessed October 21, 2021).

Kamradt-Scott, A., C. Dolea, C. Poncé, G. Rodier, M. Lamunu, P. Drury, and S. Ioos. 2018. WHO tracking mechanism for IHR additional health measures. *Lancet* 392(10161):2250–2251.

Knox, R. 2009. *Manufacturing problems with swine influenza vaccine.* https://www.npr.org/sections/health-shots/2009/07/manufacturing_problems_with_sw.html?t=1605551277283 (accessed July 6, 2021).

MacDonald, N., E. Mohsni, Y. Al-Mazrou, J. Kim Andrus, N. Arora, S. Elden, M.-Y. Madrid, R. Martin, A. Mahmoud Mustafa, H. Rees, D. Salisbury, Q. Zhao, I. Jones, C. A. Steffen, J. Hombach, K. L. O'Brien, and A. Cravioto. 2020. Global vaccine action plan lessons learned I: Recommendations for the next decade. *Vaccine* 38(33):5364–5371.

Mackenzie, J. S., M. McKinnon, and M. Jeggo. 2014. One health: From concept to practice. *Confronting Emerging Zoonoses* 163–189.

Moen, A. 2021 *Looking forward: GISRS+.* Paper presented at Influenza Preparedness and Response Health Emergencies Programme, June 22, 2021.

Monto, A. S. 2017. Moving toward improved influenza vaccines. *The Journal of Infectious Diseases* 215(4):500–502.

Moon, S., and I. Kickbusch. 2021. A pandemic treaty for a fragmented global polity. *The Lancet* 6(6):E355–E356.

Moyer, C. S. 2010. *H1N1 vaccine: what physician can do with leftover doses.* https://amednews.com/article/20100719/profession/307199943/6 (accessed December 17, 2021).

Pagliusi, S., M. Dennehy, and A. Homma. 2020. Two decades of vaccine innovations for global public good: Report of the Developing Countries' Vaccine Manufacturers Network 20th meeting, 21–23 October 2019, Rio de Janeiro, Brazil. *Vaccine* 38(36):5851–5860.

Rockman, S., K. Laurie, and I. Barr. 2020. Pandemic influenza vaccines: What did we learn from the 2009 pandemic and are we better prepared now? *Vaccines* 8(2):211.

Ruscio, B., A. Bolster, J. Bresee, A. Abelin, P. Boutet, H. Christiansen, P. Etholm, S. Desai, B. Gellin, J. Golding, M. Jit, L. Kerr, M. McKinlay, S. Kluglein, F. Lobos, S. Mathewson, M. Mazur, S. Pagliusi, P. Penttinen, D. Richardson, A. M. Ropero Alvarez, J. R. Scovitch, J. E. Seedorff, L. Shaxson, J. S. Tam, B. Taylor, N. Wairagkar, J. Watson, and A. Xeuatvongsa. 2020. Shaping meeting to explore the value of a coordinated work plan for epidemic and pandemic influenza vaccine preparedness. *Vaccine* 38(16):3179–3183.

Schroeder, K. 2018. Global challenges in seasonal influenza vaccine supply, use, and policy. *Intersect: The Stanford Journal of Science, Technology, and Society* 12(1):1–23.

Shu, Y., and J. McCauley. 2017. GISAID: Global initiative on sharing all influenza data—from vision to reality. *Euro Surveillance* 22(13):30494.

Viñuales, J., S. Moon, G. L. Moli, and G.-L. Burci. 2021. A global pandemic treaty should aim for deep prevention. *The Lancet* 397(10287):1791–1792.

WHO (World Health Organization). 2008. *International Health Regulations.* Geneva, Switzerland: World Health Organization.

WHO. 2011. *Comparative analysis of national pandemic influenza preparedness plans.* Geneva, Switzerland: World Health Organization.

WHO. 2012. *Report of the WHO pandemic influenza A (H1N1) vaccine deployment initiative.* Geneva, Switzerland: World Health Organization.

WHO. 2017. *Pandemic influenza risk management: A WHO guide to inform and harmonize national and international pandemic preparedness and response.* Geneva, Switzerland: World Health Organization. http://apps.who.int/iris/bitstream/ handle/10665/259893/ WHO-WHE-IHM-GIP-2017.1-eng.pdf?sequence=1 (accessed January 4, 2019).

WHO. 2019. *Global influenza strategy 2019–2030.* Geneva, Switzerland: World Health Organization. https://www.who.int/publications/i/item/9789241515320 (accessed October 21, 2021).

WHO. 2021 (unpublished). *Enhancing the global influenza surveillance and response system for respiratory viruses with epidemic and pandemic potential.* Draft Concept Note.

Ziegler, T., A. Mamahit, and N. J. Cox. 2018. 65 years of influenza surveillance by a World Health Organization–coordinated global network. *Influenza and Other Respiratory Viruses* 12(5):558–565.

3

Pathogen Sharing for Influenza Vaccine Production

THE ESSENTIAL NEED FOR PATHOGEN SHARING

Rapid sharing of information on pathogens is essential for effective pandemic preparedness and response (PPR). Prompt access to pathogen samples can help provide early warning about novel infectious disease threats and enable the rapid development of pathogen-specific vaccines, diagnostic tests, and medicines. Sharing viral pathogens, either the organisms themselves or their genetic sequence data, provides the means to identify vaccine targets. Modern molecular techniques allow faster development of effective vaccines, as demonstrated by the production of COVID-19 vaccines in 1 year in 2020 using platform technologies (Agrawal et al., 2021). Timely access to pathogen samples and their genetic sequence data—which can originate anywhere in the world—is therefore critical, so that organizations such as the World Health Organization (WHO) can accurately assess the risk these pathogens pose to global health, initiate the development of new medical countermeasures, and mount an appropriate international response (Elbe and Buckland-Merrett, 2017).

However, pathogen sharing has had a long and troubled history. Until roughly the early twenty-first century, it was associated with exploitative scientific and commercial practices. High-income countries (HICs), or multinational corporations in those countries, were seen as extracting resources, such as pathogen samples, from low- and middle-income countries (LMICs) to be able to manufacture and sell vaccines, diagnostics, and therapeutics while failing to share the benefits derived from those resources (Rourke, 2020).

The situation came to a brief but significant impasse in the mid-2000s during an outbreak of H5N1 influenza in much of Southeast Asia. In a 2018 workshop on Exploring Lessons Learned from a Century of Outbreaks: Readiness for 2030 at the National Academies of Sciences, Engineering, and Medicine (the National Academies), Ambassador Makarim Wibisono explained that a relatively small number of human cases of avian influenza (H5N1) in Sumatra, Indonesia, resulted in a public panic, which was heightened by the global concern about H5N1 and poultry deaths. This panic gave rise to questions about the ability of the Indonesian Ministry of Health to contain the virus (NASEM, 2019). The Indonesian government had initially complied with the Global Influenza Surveillance Network (GISN) regulations related to sharing the virus. The GISN (the precursor of the current Global Influenza Surveillance and Response System [GISRS], described in Chapter 2) required affected member countries to submit samples of their virus to WHO Collaborating Centres (WHO CCs) for identification as a potential candidate vaccine virus. The CCs then disseminate their findings to pharmaceutical companies for vaccine manufacturing. However, despite the Indonesian government's willingness to share virus samples with the GISN, it experienced great difficulty accessing the H5N1 vaccines that those samples helped produce (Rourke, 2020). When requested to provide vaccines to Indonesia, WHO responded that it did not have a process in place to supply countries directly with vaccines. In December 2006, a frustrated Indonesian government announced that it would no longer share its H5N1 virus samples with WHO CCs. Dr. Wibisono said that the Indonesian Minister of Health then pronounced the GISN process inequitable because vaccines produced from samples shared by LICs were less likely to be available to their populations (NASEM, 2019).

The 2009–2010 H1N1 pandemic also exposed several gaps and weaknesses in pathogen sharing (see Chapter 2). These reinforced that the world needed a reliable, predictable, sustainable, and timely mechanism for identifying and characterizing influenza and other viruses and sharing, or providing *access* to, these samples beyond the countries in which the viruses or sequences originated. At the same time, it also reinforced that timely sharing of viruses and associated information, such as genetic sequence data, requires attention to the *benefits* that may be derived from them. These events resulted in a major change. In May 2007, the World Health Assembly (WHA) passed a resolution to create a process for discussions that would lead to the creation of the Pandemic Influenza Preparedness (PIP) Framework, the first pathogen-specific access and benefit sharing (ABS) system, in 2011 (WHO, 2007).

According to Anne Huvos, the leader of the PIP Framework Secretariat at WHO (NASEM, 2019), the spark that drove the PIP Framework's creation process was the LMICs' loss of trust in the global system for virus sharing and access to vaccines. The LMIC governments believed that the WHO-coordinated system of virus sharing was inequitable because it failed to provide reasonable protection for their people. The initiation of the PIP Framework discussions marked the start of the trust-rebuilding process among countries. Ultimately, the process successfully facilitated virus sharing in the years after the framework was adopted.

THE CRITICAL IMPORTANCE OF ACCESS AND BENEFIT SHARING

ABS systems are designed to balance speed of access to viral information with equity in access to medical products and other assets derived from that information. This is a delicate balancing act that relies on buy-in from the governments of LMICs, HICs, and private stakeholders, such as pharmaceutical companies. Most LMICs will not support an information-sharing system for viruses that does not guarantee access to a certain percentage of vaccines. However, wealthier countries and industry are unlikely to support a system that delivers these benefits to LMICs at a significant loss of profits through mechanisms such as intellectual property (IP) waivers. Cost is a central question in the sharing of medical products and includes more than the cost of procuring vaccines themselves:

> It is not sufficient to claim these products should be shared: a mechanism to pay for and distribute them needs to be found. In some cases, charitable donations or nongovernmental organizations such as Gavi, the Vaccine Alliance, can serve this function. In others, it may be governments or drug companies that provide therapeutics or vaccines at reduced or no cost to those who need them—as did Merck, the manufacturers of the rVSV-ZEBOV Ebola vaccine, working with the U.S. Department of Health and Human Services. Nevertheless, cost is not simply a matter of the cost of producing a vaccine or therapeutic procedure. Benefit sharing may also require necessary infrastructure, such as cold chains to store and deploy products once shared, research facilities and laboratories, or basic utility systems and roadworks. (Evans et al., 2020, p. 32)

Evans and colleagues suggest that for vaccines and therapeutics, better national implementation and support for the International Health Regulations (IHR) can provide an equitable basis for sharing data and information necessary for research and later manufacturing that is negotiated ahead of time. Infrastructure investments in health care (e.g., for laboratories, roads, water, and power) before epidemics emerge can also help prevent outbreaks from becoming health emergencies.

Technology is central to this issue and often progresses more rapidly than legal frameworks. Today, the concept of pathogen sharing has expanded due to the new genetic technologies. During the 2014 Lassa outbreak in Nigeria and the 2015 Ebola outbreak in the Democratic Republic of the Congo, for example, rapid sequence sharing replaced sharing whole viruses. These trends have also accelerated during the SARS-CoV-2 pandemic but also led to complications with international collaborations.

According to Elbe and Buckland-Merrett, three main reasons remain that pathogen samples may not be shared quickly or comprehensively: concerns about acknowledgment of scientific contributions, negative economic ramifications of being identified as the source of an outbreak, and retaining ownership over IP and the monetary value of products associated with it (Elbe and Buckland-Merrett, 2017). Regardless of one's position in this balancing act, careful consideration of the components of ABS systems for pathogens, such as influenza, is essential for reliable and sustainable global delivery of vaccines in a pandemic.

EQUITY AND HUMAN RIGHTS

Infectious disease outbreaks produce at least three broad classes of benefits for individuals and communities. First, patient treatment leads to clinical data that are useful in understanding disease and improving diagnostics and surveillance of public health. Second, samples provide sequence data for surveillance technologies, diagnostics, and medical interventions. Third, experimental interventions offer both information and tangible products, such as vaccines and therapeutics (Evans et al., 2020). WHO's *Guidance for Managing Ethical Issues in Infectious Disease Outbreaks* (WHO, 2016a) suggests that all three benefits should be shared and places a "fundamental moral obligation" on researchers and other actors involved.

The discourse on the right to health and the accumulation of national and international practice and jurisprudence are gaining increasing importance in public health. They have been used as a normative tool to claim national obligations to facilitate access to essential medicines and the "determinants" of health. The right to health, as interpreted by the United Nations (UN) monitoring bodies, also has an international dimension requiring states to assist each other and not to preempt the enjoyment of the same right for the people of other countries (OHCHR, 2008). Although it would be unrealistic to argue that the right to health positively requires states to share pathogen samples and benefits, human rights considerations can be part of more detailed policy and legal considerations used to advocate cooperation or censure obstructionist behavior.

Sovereignty is one of the few influence levers that countries in the Global South have to try to create more equitable access to benefits, including vaccines. Given the reality of vaccine nationalism during the COVID-19 pandemic, it is likely that these governments will fight to retain sovereign control over pandemic strains and genetic sequence data. This reality and existing inequities must be acknowledged and addressed as ABS mechanisms are refined.

EXISTING INTERNATIONAL INSTRUMENTS FOR ABS

Four governance instruments are of particular relevance to pandemic influenza pathogen sharing and vaccine access: the IHR (revised in 2005), the UN Convention on Biological Diversity (adopted in 1992) and its Nagoya Protocol on Access to Genetic Resources and the Fair and Equitable Sharing of Benefits Arising from Their Utilization (adopted in 2010), and the PIP Framework (adopted in 2011). The impact of the latter two on vaccine preparedness and response is yet to be tested by a major influenza pandemic (see Box 3-1). Yet, over the past decade, these governance instruments' effectiveness has been increasingly challenged by technological advances. As noted, creating vaccines, therapeutics, and diagnostics now relies more heavily than ever on sharing the genetic sequence data from physical pathogen samples.

The IHR are fundamentally predicated on the concept that a coordinated multilateral response among countries is necessary to prevent and respond optimally to a pandemic threat. WHO substantively revised the IHR in 2005. Before this revision, the IHR only required case reporting and response measures justified on public health grounds for a limited number of infectious diseases, such as cholera and plague (NASEM, 2019), and influenza was not included as a reportable disease. The revised IHR now require countries to notify WHO about any disease outbreaks that could constitute a Public Health Emergency of International Concern (PHEIC). It calls on countries to develop the national capacities necessary to prevent and respond to a pandemic and to share critical information in a timely fashion. The IHR require its parties to share public information on health events that could constitute a public health emergency to enable WHO to alert the international community and to determine when to declare a PHEIC and issue consequential recommendations and guidance (Mullen et al., 2020). It does not explicitly cover sharing viruses or genetic sequence data, although some have suggested that the reference to "information" in Articles 6 through 10 can be interpreted as including sequencing data (NASEM, 2019).

As the only existing formal ABS mechanism for pathogens of pandemic potential, the PIP Framework is unique in global health governance. It emphasizes that nations, WHO, and industry have distinct and mutual responsibilities to work together to ensure that rapid sharing of potential pandemic influenza viruses and the benefits derived from this sharing are on an equal footing. WHA adopted it as a nonbinding instrument designed

BOX 3-1
Existing Instruments for Influenza Access and Benefit Sharing

The Pandemic Influenza Preparedness (PIP) Framework

The PIP Framework was unanimously adopted by the World Health Assembly on May 24, 2011, to strengthen the sharing of influenza viruses with pandemic potential and increase access to vaccines and other lifesaving supplies for countries in need.

How it works:

- Influenza vaccine manufacturers, pharmaceutical and diagnostic manufacturers, research and academic institutions, and biotech firms receive access to biological materials through the Global Influenza Surveillance and Response System (GISRS).
- In return, they must sign legally binding, negotiated agreements for benefit sharing with the World Health Organization (WHO), which can vary depending on the agreement. An agreement of this type is called a "Standard Material Transfer Agreement 2 (SMTA2)."

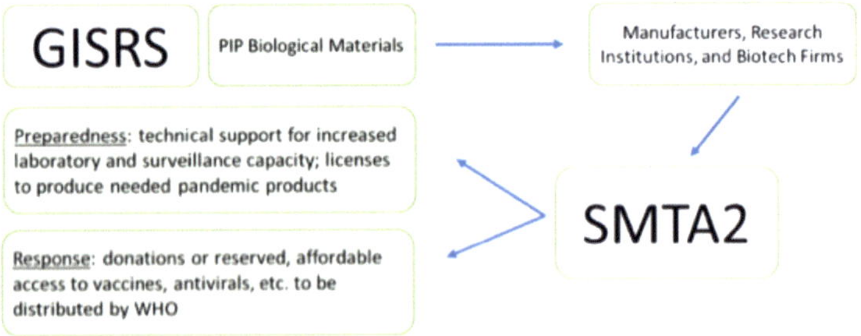

Limitations:

1. As of May 2020, 13 influenza manufacturers have signed SMTA2 agreements. This has allowed WHO to secure access to 11.3 percent of global pandemic influenza vaccine production. This can support the vaccination of priority groups in countries without influenza vaccine manufacturing capacity, but it is insufficient to cover the entire populations of LMICs.
2. Although SMTA2s between manufacturers and WHO are publicly available, transparency is limited in regard to quantifying the available vaccine supply and assessing "affordable" prices.

Funding:

3. Influenza vaccine, diagnostic, and pharmaceutical manufacturers that use GISRS make annual partnership contributions to WHO. These funds are used to strengthen pandemic preparedness capacities and to build a response fund.
4. Annual partner contributions of $28 million from industry.
   - Approximately US$28 million per year is received by WHO, of which 30 percent is reserved for the response to the next pandemic and 70 percent is used to strengthen pandemic preparedness. Total collection as of October 2020 is US$212 million.

International Health Regulations (IHR)

- The IHR, which are legally binding in 196 countries, create rights and obligations for countries, with the goal of preventing, controlling, and responding to threats of international spread of disease without unnecessarily interfering with international traffic and trade.
- Article 44 of the 2005 IHR update, on "collaboration and assistance," requires WHO, to the extent possible, to work with other international bodies and networks.

Convention on Biological Diversity (CBD) and the Nagoya Protocol

- With nearly universal sign-on, the CBD established the rights of national governments to determine access to their genetic resources, restricting access to biological resources based on mutually agreed upon terms, prior informed consent, and fair and equitable benefit-sharing practices.
- The Nagoya Protocol on Access to Genetic Resources and the Fair and Equitable Sharing of Benefits Arising from Their Utilization was signed by 129 parties, was adopted in October 2010, and went into force in 2014. As a supplementary agreement to the CBD, it provides a legal framework for effectively implementing one of the three CBD objectives: fair, equitable sharing of benefits arising from the use of genetic resources. Pathogens, including influenza, fall under this agreement—although it has not yet been determined whether genetic sequence data do.
- The Nagoya Protocol is focused on bilateral agreements but includes an option for multilateral solutions (i.e., the PIP Framework), as long as they are consistent with the objectives of the Nagoya Protocol and the CBD.

Limitations of Access and Benefit Sharing Mechanisms and Barriers to Global Coordination

There is a lack of consensus on what "utilization of genetic resources" means, what is considered a common good, and the extent to which the Nagoya Protocol applies to pandemic influenza viruses (under the PIP Framework):

Type of Pathogen	Falls Under the PIP Framework	Falls Under the Nagoya Protocol	Coordinated by an Existing Multilateral Mechanism
Influenza viruses with human pandemic potential	Yes	Yes	Yes
Seasonal influenza	No	Yes	No
Genetic sequence data (Influenza)	No	Not clear	No
Other pathogens	No	Yes	No
Genetic sequence data (other pathogens)	No	Not clear	No

SOURCE: Adapted from Huvos et al., 2020.

to govern pandemic influenza pathogen sharing and the distribution of vaccines, diagnostics, and therapeutics using an innovative model that engages industry through prenegotiated contracts (WHO, 2011). It sets the amount of real-time supply under contracts that companies agree to provide for a pandemic and explicitly requires industry to pay an annual fixed partnership contribution of $28 million, which was originally calculated as covering 50 percent of the operating costs of the GISRS. (Chapter 5 discusses GISRS funding further.)

However, the scope of the PIP Framework is restricted to influenza viruses of pandemic potential. In 2016, an expert review found that the PIP Framework is "a bold and innovative tool for pandemic influenza preparedness, is being well implemented, and that the principle of the PIP Framework of placing virus sharing and benefit sharing on an equal footing remains relevant today" (WHO, 2016b, p. 12). Its implementation has resulted in greater confidence and predictability in global capacity to respond to an influenza pandemic. Its success is partially due to regular engagement by WHO and its member states with key stakeholders, including industry and civil society. However, key issues remain, including how genetic sequence data should be handled, whether the Framework could be expanded to include *seasonal* influenza, and whether it could be used as a model for sharing of other pathogens.

Given the flexibility and agility of GISRS to respond to COVID-19, WHO is assessing the opportunities to expand GISRS so that it addresses other respiratory viruses with epidemic and pandemic potential more regularly and systematically (see Chapter 2). "GISRS+" would build from the influenza backbone to provide an integrated platform for the surveillance and monitoring of respiratory viruses and serve as a global alert mechanism for the emergence of novel respiratory viruses. In an unpublished communication to the National Academies, the WHO Influenza Group also noted[1] an opportunity to create a new ABS system that establishes fair and equitable benefit sharing taking into account (1) timeliness of access to benefits, (2) affordability to the end user, and (3) quantity of benefits shared. It stated that any new system should incorporate the "real time" dimension of access to pandemic products by WHO; maintain the status of vaccine supply from manufacturers as largely (80 percent) donations so that WHO can continue to donate these supplies to countries based on need; and preserve WHO's 10 percent access to future pandemic vaccine production in real time.

The Nagoya Protocol under the Convention on Biological Diversity (CBD) spells out in detail the general benefit-sharing provisions of the CBD.

[1] Considerations and input from the WHO Influenza Group to address questions from the National Academies Global Coordination Study Working Group on Pathogen Sharing, May 2021.

The CBD codified the principle of national sovereignty over biological and genetic resources, which has increasingly included pathogens, through national practice. The CBD and Nagoya Protocol's provisions were developed as a reaction to IP debates in the 1990s. The protocol was not initially designed with public health in mind and did not explicitly consider the pandemic context. Under the protocol, a pathogen with pandemic potential is viewed in the context of national sovereignty; the approach is based on negotiated country-to-country two-party agreements as the basis for sharing genetic materials and the benefits resulting from their use. It recognizes the sovereignty of a country to determine how its genetic resources are used, requires that access to genetic resources must have the prior informed consent of the effective or originating country, and specifies that those resources can only be accessed by negotiating mutually agreed terms that include benefit sharing.

In May 2019, the WHA requested that the WHO Director-General prepare a report on the public health implications of implementation of the Nagoya Protocol. In response, the Office of WHO's Chief Scientist surveyed all key internal stakeholders, including the Secretariat of the PIP Framework, focal points for the IHR, and the food safety and communicable disease teams. The WHO Secretariat also contacted member states and other stakeholders, including the Secretariat of the Convention on Biological Diversity; UN agencies, funds, and programs such as the Food and Agriculture Organization; other international agencies, such as the World Organisation for Animal Health (OIE); and civil society and public-sector entities.

The resulting report, *The Public Health Implications of Implementation of the Nagoya Protocol* (WHO, 2021a), was released in January 2021. The overall view in survey responses was that pathogen sharing is positive for public health if well regulated and transparent and the benefits are agreed upon and shared among both the data generators and receivers. Similarly, there was convergence that pathogen sharing enables multijurisdictional and international outbreak investigations and improves the quality of laboratory surveillance. This can provide major benefits in relation to R&D; diagnostic test validation in public health emergencies; transfer of technologies and expertise, including opportunities for laboratories to work with pathogens to which they would not ordinarily have access; and due recognition and protections for the source provider. Respondents in general noted that pathogen sharing is easier when bilateral agreements already exist between institutions and the researchers know and trust each other. Most respondents also indicated that genetic sequence data should be differentiated from physical sample sharing. Differences that were highlighted included risks of handling physical samples; the broader potential for sharing genetic sequence data; and the logistical differences related to biosafety and biosecurity, cold-chain storage equipment, qualified personnel, correct certificates, and adequate transportation. Sharing genetic sequence data is often more complex because of the difference in scale and multiple ways of sharing, altering, and resharing. Issues of public availability for genetic sequence data are more concerned with ensuring appropriate credit for the work and data privacy issues.

The report also raised two broad challenges for human pathogen sharing. First, respondents noted an absence of a harmonized system across countries and unclear domestic guidelines and that this gap is exacerbated by recipient laboratories that are not aware of, do not have time to understand, or do not comply with ABS arrangements. Second, lack of awareness of the Nagoya Protocol and its requirements and the individualized implementation mechanisms unique to each state party to the protocol add complications. More general concerns include bureaucratic delays; overlapping, conflicting, or unclear processes for customs clearance and other regulatory requirements; lack of international couriers qualified to handle shipments; multiple approval levels for sharing with external parties; lengthy negotiations; lack of procedures for unified national biosafety regulations and harmonization across jurisdictions; language barriers; and restrictions regarding dual use (WHO, 2021a).

Article 4(4) of the Nagoya Protocol stipulates that

> Where a specialized international access and benefit-sharing instrument applies that is consistent with, and does not run counter to, the objectives of the Convention and this Protocol, this Protocol does not apply for the Party or Parties to the specialized instrument in respect of the specific genetic resource covered by and for the purpose of the specialized instrument. (Convention on Biological Diversity, 2011)

In addition, under Article 8(b) of the protocol, parties shall

> pay due regard to cases of present or imminent emergencies that threaten or damage human ... health, as determined nationally or internationally. Parties may take into consideration the need for expeditious access to genetic resources and expeditious fair and equitable sharing of benefits arising out of the use of such genetic resources....

These two provisions appear to allow for a special international instrument to address a need for rapid pathogen sharing during a pandemic.

BARRIERS AND GAPS THAT AFFECT ABS FOR INFLUENZA

Each of the four governance instruments discussed above has gaps as well as some provisions that establish barriers to ABS.

The IHR: The IHR gaps could pose barriers to pathogen sharing. The challenge is to operationalize collaboration under Article 44, which requires countries to collaborate and assist each other in meeting their obligations and WHO to collaborate with state parties to the same end. What is missing is an explicit definition of what the "obligations" for member states and WHO are. Article 44 encourages states to collaborate "to the extent possible" to detect and respond to potential public health emergencies and share "technical, logistical, financial, and legal support to help other states implement the IHR" (Fischer et al., 2011). However, donor nations have been slow to distribute comprehensive assistance packages to help resource-constrained countries achieve the core IHR capacities. One reason is that the scope of this challenge is tremendous and requires strengthening public health surveillance and response systems, producing a trained health workforce, creating infrastructure and tools, and developing cross-sector communications and coordination. A standard global blueprint to accomplish these competencies is lacking, so national public health authorities must map their own courses. Just figuring out where to start can be daunting (Fischer et al., 2011). Perhaps more important is competing priorities: both donors and domestic governments find it hard to prioritize strengthening IHR core competencies over more immediate health needs, such as combating the epidemics of HIV, TB, and malaria.

Although the IHR do not specifically mention genetic sequence data, it would be possible for the WHA to interpret Articles 6–10 to include that as part of the "information" or "data" that states parties are required to submit to WHO or share among themselves.

The PIP Framework: The Framework's gaps also could obstruct pathogen sharing. As already noted, its scope is restricted to pandemic influenza. Despite suggestions that it be expanded to encompass seasonal influenza, discussions of this at WHO have been inconclusive. The pharmaceutical industry also opposes this. The consequences are the absence of benefit-sharing provisions for seasonal influenza viruses (WHO, 2016b). If the framework were expanded to include seasonal influenza, the benefits to be shared would need to be more clearly defined. The Third World Network (TWN) has noted that seasonal and pandemic influenza have different dynamics—for seasonal influenza, countries decide to either use or not use vaccines, but during a pandemic, all nations want them. The Framework also does not specifically encompass genetic sequence data in its definition of what is covered by its benefit-sharing provisions.

Contemporary global governance structures, such as the multilateral commitments under the PIP Framework, have yet to be tested by a serious influenza pandemic (NASEM, 2019). How would benefit-sharing function, and is it vulnerable in such circumstances? Stronger multilateral commitments could help. However, the PIP Framework also has no requirements for developing its norms, no oversight beyond the advisory role played by the PIP Advisory Group, and no reminder for governments of the commitments they have undertaken. Vaccine "nationalism," as expressed in advance purchase agreements and export controls, may undermine the operations of benefit distribution during a pandemic. A gap may also occur between when PIP partner distributions are activated and contributions must be received. Furthermore, even when donations are realized, what distribution of vaccines and other products is equitable? Under COVAX, the "vaccine pillar" of the Access to COVID-19 Tools (ACT) Accelerator, which is a global collaboration to accelerate development, production, and equitable access to COVID-19 tests, treatments, and vaccines, the target is 20 percent of the population in a receiving country. Under the PIP Framework, partner contributions can also be allocated for building manufacturing capacity, but the intended financing for this purpose may be insufficient.

The CBD and the Nagoya Protocol: These instruments can be barriers in themselves; they present a strong tension between sharing viruses for public health reasons and sharing other benefits for countries that provide biological information about disease organisms. The Nagoya Protocol's strong emphasis on benefit sharing is a potent tool to ensure ABS, but public health emergencies suggest that benefit sharing be balanced by pathogen sharing.

The extent to which the Nagoya Protocol is applicable to the pandemic influenza context is an open question. Many aspects of the protocol are not necessarily incompatible with the IHR and PIP Framework and the specific needs of global health security. However, conflicting principles and severe operational incompatibilities exist. In a pandemic, responses must happen quickly over hours, days, or weeks, but negotiating bilateral agreements under Nagoya can take much longer. As noted, one of the more common concerns about its compatibility with the more urgent needs for public health threats is the potential for delays in virus sharing. In 2021, the WHO Director-General prepared a report for its executive board where he discussed how virus sharing delays can negatively impact the vaccine virus selection process (WHO, 2021a). The GISAID argues that it is important to not only think of the impacts of the Nagoya Protocol in the future but also reflect on its past consequences (GISAID, 2019). With a reported 6–9-month delay in accessing influenza samples (IFPMA, 2019), the suitability of bilateral negotiations in a pandemic setting where viruses may spread quickly is highly questionable (WHO, 2021a).

National sovereignty can also be a barrier for influenza and other respiratory pathogens with pandemic potential. Industry, TWN, and other nongovernmental organizations have noted that if an entire society is affected by a pandemic, as with COVID-19, a new procedural paradigm for decision making in this context is needed. Country-by-country negotiations are likely to get in the way (Correa, 2021; TWN, 2020). As COVID-19 has shown, vaccine nationalism can be counter to public health needs and undermine the positive aspects of pathogen and benefit sharing (Abbas, 2020). Weak leadership and politics can also pose barriers. Considerations of equity and the broader human right to health could be balanced against the considerations and procedural requirements of the Nagoya Protocol. Fragmentation, or lack of effective global coordination, can also be a barrier. Other forums and accountability mechanisms could be used to achieve the benefit sharing sought under Nagoya. ABS may fall under different legal regimes that are not always easy to reconcile, including considerations on biodiversity, the IHR, trade law, biosecurity due to concerns about dual use of pathogens, and human rights.

HOW HAS THE "COVID-19 LENS" CHANGED THE WAY GOVERNMENTS, ORGANIZATIONS, AND INSTITUTIONS LOOK AT ABS INSTRUMENTS?

These governance instruments represent a unique influenza "ecosystem" of pre-existing global networks, standards, and practices. This ecosystem was largely not activated for the COVID-19 pandemic; the IHR did not cover sample, genetic sequence, or benefit sharing; little attention was paid to the Nagoya Protocol in the extreme situation posed by COVID-19 largely because the virus' fast and wide spread bypassed the protocol's sovereignty-based foundation; and the PIP Framework was not applicable because its scope is restricted to pandemic influenza (and no similar ABS mechanism exists for other pathogens with pandemic potential). Instead, COVID-19 vaccine development has been dominated by unilateral or bilateral decision making by national governments and companies and the support of ad hoc and newly created mechanisms, such as the ACT Accelerator and COVAX; the intensification of existing mechanisms, such as the GISAID Initiative, a public–private partnership; and the proliferation of scientific collaborations and publications by members of the global scientific community.

Initiatives such as the U.S. Operation Warp Speed (described in Chapter 4) have demonstrated the advantages of an approach where pharmaceutical companies that are supported by national funding can respond quickly using multiple and often new technologies to produce vaccines rapidly. However, it has also shown that rich countries, as usual, receive vaccines ahead of all others, distribution is largely subject to current political priorities, and provision of viruses and genetic sequence data is not predictable or necessarily reliable. Furthermore, it spotlighted ABS issues with new mechanisms advanced or proposed, including COVAX, WHO's BioHub System, and discussions of IP waivers and a potential pandemic treaty. In many respects, these discussions are being driven by the same issues underlying the urgent discussions after the emergence of H5N1 influenza in 1997 and 2003, SARS in 2003, and Ebola in West Africa in 2014. As discussed, some of these events led to the adoption of the revised IHR in 2005 and the PIP Framework in 2011.

Three evolving initiatives are of particular relevance to ABS for pathogens with pandemic potential. First, in May 2021, the Swiss Confederation and WHO signed a memorandum of understanding to launch the first WHO BioHub Facility as part of the new WHO BioHub System, which was first announced in November 2020. This will be based out of Spiez, Switzerland, and its purpose will be to enhance the rapid sharing of viruses and other pathogens globally between laboratories and partners. It will be a center for the safe receiving, sequencing, storage, and preparation of biological materials for distribution to other laboratories. These materials will be used to inform risk assessments and sustain global preparedness against SARS-CoV-2 and other emerging pathogens. The BioHub System is intended "to address the fact that, currently, most pathogen sharing is done bilaterally between countries and on an ad hoc basis, which can be slow, and leave some countries without access to the benefits and tools." It is intended to enable member states to share biological materials with and via the BioHub under pre-agreed conditions and in compliance with biosafety, biosecurity, and other applicable regulations to ensure timeliness and predictability in response activities (WHO, 2021b,c). WHO plans to broaden BioHub for the use of biological materials by qualified entities—such as manufacturers—to develop medical products for fair allocation to member countries. WHO is running a pilot phase using SARS-CoV-2 to test the feasibility and operational arrangements for sharing such materials with BioHub. It is intended to expand to other pathogens, and, in 2022, to connect partners with other repositories and laboratory networks. However, the proposal has been criticized by some, such as TWN and South Centre, for lacking specific reference to equitable sharing of benefits, a concept that is an integral part of the discourse on biodiversity law and policy (Hammond, 2021; South Centre, 2021).

Second, much recent discussion and debate has taken place on IP waivers. The proposed Agreement on the Trade-Related Intellectual Property Rights (TRIPS) waiver resulted from concerns about the impact of IP barriers on the scale-up of manufacturing of lifesaving tools, including vaccines, for COVID-19. World Trade Organization (WTO) members can invoke a waiver of certain IP rights due to exceptional global crises. In October 2020, India and South Africa proposed that the WTO allow all countries the legal right under international trade rules to choose not to grant or enforce patents and other IP related to COVID-19 drugs, vaccines, diagnostics, and other technologies and materials until widespread vaccination is in place globally and the majority of the world population has developed an immunity (Menezes, 2021). This proposal gained momentum, and 64 countries had cosponsored it as of September 2021. However, vaccine patenting involves complex issues. For example, some of the main platform technologies for COVID-19 vaccines had already been used for previous vaccines and are under patent control. A large portfolio of IP also exists on mRNA technology, although Moderna has elected not to enforce its patents during the pandemic.

The perspectives on IP waivers are, as might reasonably be anticipated, very different for governments, civil society organizations (CSOs), and industry. In a 2021 research paper, the South Centre represented the views of CSOs, arguing that to be in line with the May 2020 WHA-approved "COVID-19 Response" Resolution (WHA 73.1), WHO member states need to recognize COVID-19 responses as a global public good and "any unjustified obstacles must be removed, and TRIPS flexibilities should be strengthened" (Menezes, 2021). The UN General Assembly also passed resolutions emphasizing the need to rapidly scale up manufacturing and strengthen supply chains for efficient, timely, fair, transparent, and equitable access to and distribution of diagnostics, drugs, and COVID-19 vaccines. The president of Costa Rica proposed the COVID-19 Technology Access Pool early in the pandemic for voluntary, nonexclusive licensing. It was received with apparent enthusiasm, but it collapsed without widespread buy-in. Its failure to attract support underscores how voluntary mechanisms depend on the participation and direct collaboration of "Big Pharma" to be successful.

The industry perspective, as represented by the International Federation of Pharmaceutical Manufacturers & Associations (IFPMA), in May 2021 expressed disappointment with the U.S. decision to support an IP waiver as "the simple but the wrong answer to what is a complex problem." In IFPMA's words,

> Waiving patents of COVID-19 vaccines will not increase production nor provide practical solutions needed to battle this global health crisis. On the contrary, it is likely to lead to disruption; while distracting from addressing the real challenges in scaling up production and distribution of COVID-19 vaccines globally: namely elimination of trade barriers, addressing bottlenecks in supply chains and scarcity of raw materials and ingredients in the supply chain, and a willingness by rich countries to start sharing doses with poor countries. (IFPMA, 2021)

Thus, industry opposition to imposed IP waivers is clear. Such waivers could also act as a disincentive for vaccine development and manufacturing or result in manufacturing that is not up to standards.

Third, as described in Chapter 2, discussions are ongoing about developing a new "pandemic treaty" that would address the gaps in existing governance instruments. It could articulate key principles, roles, and responsibilities for sharing viruses and benefits and potentially establish penalties for failure to comply. However, a global treaty negotiation is likely to require many years because so many constituencies, including civil society, industry, national and international health organizations, and North- and South-associated country groupings, would have to be involved. Such negotiations would also require consistent and committed political leadership that supports a strong multilateral approach that could bring together all interests. At the WHA in May 2021, over two dozen countries signed on to support a global treaty, while the United States, Russia, and China held off. This conversation will be continued in a special session of the WHA in November 2021 (Furlong, 2021). Nevertheless, a new treaty represents an opportunity to incorporate earlier diplomatic gains and agreed-upon principles in the PIP Framework into a new long-term multilateral agreement.

KEY FINDINGS AND CONCLUSIONS

- The PIP Framework is built on the needs for transparency, equity, efficiency, and accountability of countries, industry, and WHO. Beyond access to vaccines and medicines at reduced prices, other essential benefits can include capacity building, training, and publications.
- The PIP Framework's ability to ensure the availability of vaccines and antiviral medications under pandemic conditions and to distribute them equitably remains untested.
- There is a major gap regarding sharing genetic sequence data due to uncertainty about whether it falls under the PIP Framework, the CBD, and the Nagoya Protocol. It is still necessary for the PIP Framework to be modified to include genetic sequence data.
- While it remains theoretically possible for the PIP Framework to be expanded to include seasonal influenza, other viruses, and genetic sequence data, it does not appear to be a realistic option to scale up the pandemic influenza–specific framework to encompass other respiratory pathogens with pandemic potential.
- The underlying core principles of the PIP Framework remain highly relevant and should be incorporated into a pandemic treaty or other future international instrument. These principles include (1) giving equal weight to sharing of viruses and of benefits, which are equally important, (2) sharing responsibility and accountability among countries, WHO, and the private sector (although, under the framework, both industry and civil society operate through member states), (3) recognizing that responding to country needs is fundamentally important, particulary for LMICs, and (4) ensuring benefits flow multilaterally and not bilaterally.

- Secondary PIP Framework issues include the specific ways that it is implemented. These can be modified and negotiated for future multilateral agreements covering ABS for pathogens with pandemic potential.
- Delays in sharing samples, sequences, and information have serious implications for delaying a pandemic response. Every player—including National Influenza Centres, countries, vaccine manufacturers, and WHO—can have both immediate self-serving and collaborative behavior. It is therefore critical to encourage and enable rapid sharing and characterization of samples.
- Seasonal pathogen sharing has increasingly been negatively impacted by the Nagoya Protocol, resulting in the need to choose alternate virus strains for vaccines. In a potential pandemic situation, this behavior in sharing viruses and associated information could have very serious implications for delaying a pandemic response.
- A new agreement should address and resolve issues raised by the Nagoya Protocol for sharing influenza viruses and other pathogens with pandemic potential, including genetic sequence data.

REFERENCES

Abbas, M. Z. 2020. *Practical implications of "vaccine nationalism": A short-sighted and risky approach in response to COVID-19*. South Centre Research 124. Geneva, Switzerland: South Centre. https://www.southcentre.int/research-paper-124-november-2020 (accessed December 19, 2021).

Agrawal, G., R. Hermann., R. Poetes, M. Steinmann, and M. Moller. 2021. *Fast-forward: Will the speed of COVID-19 vaccine development reset industry norms?* https://www.mckinsey.com/industries/life-sciences/our-insights/fast-forward-will-the-speed-of-covid-19-vaccine-development-reset-industry-norms (accessed December 19, 2021).

Convention on Biological Diversity. 2011. *Text of the Nagoya Protocol: Article 4. Relationship with international agreements and instruments*. https://www.cbd.int/abs/text/articles/?sec=abs-04 (accessed June 4, 2021).

Correa, C. M. 2021. Vaccination inequalities and the role of the multilateral system. *South Views No. 224*. The South Centre, 19 July, 2021. https://www.southcentre.int/wp-content/uploads/2021/07/SouthViews-Correa.pdf (accessed October 23, 2021).

Elbe, S., and G. Buckland-Merrett. 2017. Data, disease and diplomacy: GISAID's innovative contribution to global health. *Global Challenges* 1(1):33–46.

Evans, N. G., K. Hills, K., and A. C. Levine. 2020. How should the WHO guide access and benefit sharing during infectious disease outbreaks? *AMA Journal of Ethics* 22:E28–E35.

Fischer, E., J. K. Rebecca, and S. Kornblet. 2011. *The International Health Regulations (2005): Surveillance and response in an era of globalization*. Washington, DC: Stimson Center.

Furlong, A. 2021. *U.S. succeeds in efforts to delay pandemic treaty*. *Politico*, May 25, 2021. https://www.politico.eu/article/us-succeeds-in-efforts-to-delay-pandemic-treaty (accessed October 21, 2021).

GISAID. 2019. *GISAID's comments on the WHO Report of the Public Health Implications of Implementation of the Nagoya Protocol.* https://www.gisaid.org/references/statements-clarifications/who-report-on-the-public-health-implications-of-nagoya-protocol-13-may-2019 (accessed October 23, 2021).

Hammond, E. 2021. *Questions swirl about proposed WHO pathogen collection: Effort to "shortcut" the Nagoya Protocol raises fairness and equity and other issues.* Third World Network Briefing Paper. https://www.twn.my/title2/briefing_papers/twn/Questions%20about%20proposed%20WHO%20pathogen%20collection%20Jan2021%20Hammond.pdf (accessed July 19, 2021).

Huvos, A., S. A. Solomon, and C. Nannini. 2020. The pandemic influenza preparedness framework as an access and benefit sharing mechanism. In *Viral sovereignty and technology transfer: The changing global system for sharing pathogens for public health research*, pp. 193–204. Cambridge, UK: Cambridge University Press. https://www.cambridge.org/core/books/abs/viral-sovereignty-and-technology-transfer/pandemic-influenza-preparedness-framework-as-an-access-and-benefit-sharing-mechanism/535884BE78E4F5AE1D2A882F2D806CB1 (accessed October 23, 2021).

IFPMA (International Federation of Pharmaceutical Manufacturers & Associations). 2019. *Tackling global health challenges.* https://www.ifpma.org/subtopics/public-health-implications-of-the-implementation-of-the-nagoya-protocol (accessed July 19, 2021).

IFPMA. 2021. *IFPMA Statement on WTO TRIPS intellectual property waiver.* https://www.ifpma.org/resource-centre/ifpma-statement-on-wto-trips-intellectual-property-waiver (accessed October 23, 2021).

Menezes, H. Z. d. 2021. *The TRIPS waiver proposal: An urgent measure to expand access to the COVID-19 vaccines.* South Centre Research Paper 129. Geneva, Switzerland: South Centre. https://www.southcentre.int/research-paper-129-march-2021 (accessed December 19, 2021).

Mullen, L. P. C., Gosten, L. O., Cicero, A., and Nuzzo, J. B. 2020. An analysis of International Health Regulations Emergency Committees and Public Health Emergency of International Concern Designations. *BMJ Global Health.* https://www.centerforhealthsecurity.org/our-work/publications/an-analysis-of-international-health-regulations-emergency-committees-and-public-health-emergency-of-international-concern-designations (accessed October 23, 2021).

NASEM (National Academies of Sciences, Engineering, and Medicine). 2019. *Exploring lessons learned from a century of outbreaks: Readiness for 2030: Proceedings of a workshop.* Washington, DC: The National Academies Press.

OHCHR (Office of the United Nations High Commissioner for Human Rights). 2008. *The right to health.* Fact Sheet 31. The Human Rights Fact Sheet Series. The Office of the United Nations High Commissioner for Human Rights. https://www.ohchr.org/Documents/Publications/Factsheet31.pdf (accessed October 23, 2021).

Rourke, M. F. 2020. Restricting access to pathogen samples and epidemiological data: A not-so-brief history of "viral sovereignty" and the mark it left on the world. *Infectious Diseases in the New Millennium: Legal and Ethical Challenges* 82:167–191.

South Centre. 2021. *Ensuring a sustainable and resilient response to COVID-19 and emerging infectious diseases through local production.* https://www.southcentre.int/un-hlpf-side-event-6-july-2021 (accessed October 23, 2021).

TWN (Third World Network). 2020. *South voices concerns over "vaccine nationalism" amid COVID-19.* https://www.twn.my/title2/wto.info/2020/ti200807.htm (accessed October 23, 2021).

WHO (World Health Organization). 2007. *WHA60.28 Pandemic influenza preparedness: Sharing of influenza viruses and access to vaccines and other benefits.* Geneva, Switzerland: World Health Organization.

WHO. 2011. *Pandemic influenza preparedness: Framework for the sharing of influenza viruses and access to vaccines and other benefits*. Geneva, Switzerland: World Health Organization.

WHO. 2016a. *Guidance for managing ethical issues in infection disease outbreaks*. Geneva, Switzerland: World Health Organization.

WHO. 2016b. *Review of the Pandemic Influenza Preparedness Framework*. Geneva, Switzerland: World Health Organization. https://apps.who.int/gb/ebwha/pdf_files/WHA70/A70_17-en.pdf (accessed October 23, 2021).

WHO. 2021a. *The public health implications of implementation of the Nagoya Protocol, Report by the Director-General*. Geneva, Switzerland: World Health Organization.

WHO. 2021b. *WHO and Switzerland launch global BioHub for pathogen storage, sharing and analysis*. Geneva, Switzerland: World Health Organization. https://www.who.int/news/item/24-05-2021-who-and-switzerland-launch-global-biohub-for-pathogen-storage-sharing-and-analysis (accessed June 4, 2021).

WHO. 2021c. *The WHO BioHub system for preparedness and response to epidemics and pandemics: Concept note*. Geneva, Switzerland: World Health Organization. https://cdn.who.int/media/docs/default-source/2021-dha-docs/210617_whobiohubconceptnote_brochure-(1).pdf?sfvrsn=5e5a06f3_1percentdownload=truhttps://cdn.who.int/media/docs/default-source/2021-dha-docs/210617_whobiohubconceptnote_brochure-(1).pdf?sfvrsn=5e5a06f3_1percentdownload=tru (accessed October 23, 2021).

4

Technology and Manufacturing Partnerships

PLATFORM TECHNOLOGIES IN THE COVID-19 ERA

Industry partnerships for platform technologies (technologies used as a base on which other applications, processes, or technologies are developed) forged during the COVID-19 pandemic are poised to offer a disruptive moment,[1] including for those used for influenza vaccines. COVID-19 has accelerated the shift toward messenger RNA (mRNA) and recombinant vaccines. In its May 4, 2021 earnings call, Pfizer reported 2021 sales projections that estimated that its COVID-19 vaccine—"Comirnaty"—would generate 1-year sales that far exceeded those of any pharmaceutical product in history (LaMattina, 2021). Unsurprisingly, Pfizer is looking to harness the mRNA platform technology advancements to develop a more effective influenza vaccine. The company's chief scientific officer and president of research and development (R&D), Michael Dolsten, informed investors that Pfizer will start clinical trials for its influenza mRNA vaccine during the third quarter of 2021 (LaMattina, 2021).

The COVID-19 pandemic has also helped to attract and drive new players into the vaccine market. Only 14 percent of organizations involved in pandemic-related product development had commercialized vaccines, although many had experience in developing vaccines against Zika virus, Ebola virus, Middle East respiratory syndrome coronavirus (MERS-CoV), SARS-CoV-1, H1N1 influenza, and various other diseases (Chagar et al.,

[1] Techopedia. https://www.techopedia.com/definition/3411/platform (accessed January 14, 2022).

2021). More than 20 COVID-19 vaccines are being produced around the world. Figure 4-1 depicts the production locations. Table 4-1 lists the vaccine manufacturers by platform.

About two-thirds of the current COVID-19 vaccines in the pipeline rely on established technologies such as protein subunit vaccines, nonreplicating viral vectors, and inactivated viruses. The remaining use newer technologies—including mRNA and adenovirus vectors—that could serve as "plug-and-play" platforms for vaccines against other pathogens. To confer protection against infectious diseases, mRNA vaccines introduce a piece of mRNA that corresponds to a protein or a component thereof in the virus, inducing cells in the body to produce that protein, triggering an immune response that produces antibodies against the protein that persist and can prevent infection and serious illness after exposure to the target virus. COVID-19 vaccines based on the adenovirus vector technology trigger an immune response using a nonreplicating viral vector that delivers the genetic code for the spike protein on the surface of the SARS-CoV-2 virus. Both mRNA and adenovirus approaches to vaccine development have been studied for other emerging viruses, including Zika and MERS. Zabdeno, a vaccine against *Zaire ebolavirus* developed using adenovirus vector technology, was licensed by the European Medicines Agency in 2020.

Funding from a range of agencies and organizations—including the U.S. Department of Defense, the U.S. Biomedical Advanced Research and Development Authority (BARDA), the U.S. National Institutes of Health (NIH), the United Kingdom, and the Coalition for Epidemic Preparedness Innovations (CEPI)—has been instrumental in developing the technologies

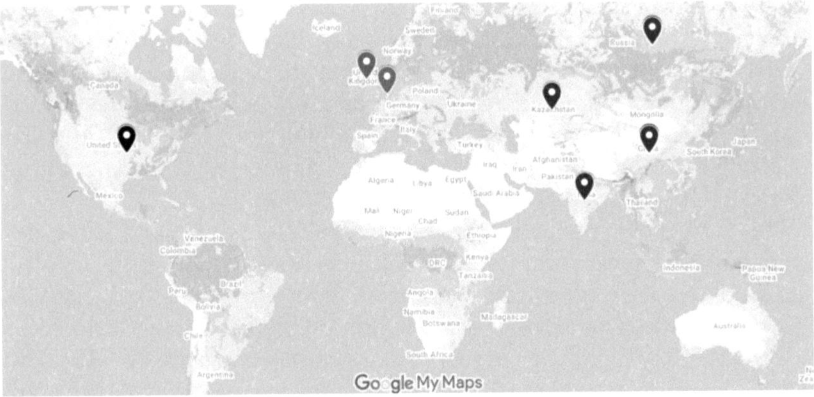

FIGURE 4-1 Global landscape of some of the COVID-19 vaccine production locations in March 2021.
SOURCE: Based on data from the COVID-19 Vaccine Manufacturing Potential map, with data through March 2021. http://vaxmap.org (accessed March 31, 2021).

TABLE 4-1 Approved Vaccines, Manufacturers, and Platforms

Vaccine Type	Name	Developer	Country
Nonreplicating viral vector	COVID-19 Vaccine Oxford/AstraZeneca (AZD1222)	BARDA, OWS	United Kingdom
Inactivated vaccine	BBIBP-CorV	Beijing Institute of Biological Products; China National Pharmaceutical Group (Sinopharm)	China
Inactivated vaccine	Covaxin (BBV152)	Bharat Biotech, Indian Council of Medical Research; Ocugen, National Institute of Virology	India
Inactivated vaccine	WIBP-CorV	Wuhan Institute of Biological Products; China National Pharmaceutical Group (Sinopharm)	China
Inactivated vaccine	CoviVac	Chumakov Federal Scientific Center for Research and Development of Immune and Biological Products	Russia
Inactivated vaccine	QazVac (QazCovid-in)	Research Institute for Biological Safety Problems	Kazakhstan
Inactivated vaccine	KCONVAC	Minhai Biotechnology Co.; Kangtai Biological Products Co. Ltd.	China
Inactivated vaccine (formalin with alum adjuvant)	CoronaVac	Sinovac, PT Bio Farma, Instituto Butantan	China
mRNA-based vaccine	Comirnaty (BNT162b2)	Pfizer, BioNTech; Fosun Pharma	United States
mRNA-based vaccine	Moderna COVID19 Vaccine (mRNA-1273)	Moderna, BARDA, NIAID	United States
Nonreplicating viral vector	COVID-19 Vaccine Janssen (JNJ-78436735; Ad26.COV2.S)	Janssen Vaccines (Johnson & Johnson)	The Netherlands, United States
Peptide vaccine	EpiVacCorona	Federal Budgetary Research Institution State Research Center of Virology and Biotechnology, Rospotrebnadzor	Russia
Recombinant adenovirus vaccine (rAd26 and rAd5)/ nonreplicating viral vector	Sputnik V	Gamaleya Research Institute, Acellena Contract Drug Research and Development	Russia

continued

TABLE 4-1 Continued

Vaccine Type	Name	Developer	Country
Recombinant adenovirus vaccine (rAd26)/ nonreplicating viral vector	Sputnik Light	Gamaleya Research Institute, Acellena Contract Drug Research and Development	Russia
Recombinant vaccine	ZF2001	Anhui Zhifei Longcom Biopharmaceutical, Institute of Microbiology of the Chinese Academy of Sciences	China, Uzbekistan
Recombinant vaccine (adenovirus type 5 vector)/ nonreplicating viral vector	Convidicea (PakVac, Ad5-nCoV)	CanSino Biologics	China
Protein subunit	CIGB-66	Center for Genetic Engineering and Biotechnology	Thailand
Protein subunit	MVC-COV1901	Medigen Vaccine Biologics Corp.	Taiwan
Nonreplicating viral vector	Covishield	Serum Institute of India (Oxford/AstraZeneca formulation)	India
Inactivated vaccine	COVID-19 inactivated	Shifa Pharmed Industrial	Iran
mRNA	TAK-919	Takeda (Moderna formulation)	Japan
DNA	ZyCoV-D	Zydus Cadila	India

NOTE: BARDA = Biomedical Advanced Research and Development Authority; NIAID = National Institute of Allergy and Infectious Diseases; OWS = Operation Warp Speed.
SOURCE: Airfinity or the COVID19 Vaccine Tracker, https://covid19.trackvaccines.org/vaccines/approved (accessed September 30, 2021). Data through September 2021.

used in new vaccines (Sabin-Aspen Vaccine Science and Policy Group, 2021). Manufacturers of vaccines using mRNA and protein subunits will likely be incentivized to shift to new antigenic targets, including for influenza, to continue capitalizing on the new technology developed for COVID-19. This represents a potentially transformative inflection point in the influenza vaccine manufacturing landscape. Certain technologies supported by BARDA for pandemic influenza—mRNA (Moderna), adenovirus 26 (Janssen), recombinant protein (Sanofi), and nanoparticle (Novavax)—were adapted for SARS-COV-2 with support from the U.S. government and ultimately granted emergency use authorization by the

U.S. Food and Drug Administration. Although it would require substantial R&D followed by clinical trials, this underscores the potential to transfer platform technologies for pandemic influenza vaccines and therapeutics to other emerging infectious diseases and vice versa (Newland et al., 2021).

NEW INDUSTRY PARTNERSHIPS DURING COVID-19

The launch of these new platform technologies during the COVID-19 pandemic has led to a plethora of new industry partnerships, many forged among companies that have traditionally been in direct competition. In the words of the Sabin-Aspen Vaccine Science and Policy Group (2019, p. 19), "Nothing in recent times has showcased the payoff of basic science investment as much as COVID-19 vaccines—a decades-long overnight success story that drew on years of earlier research to confront a devastating new virus." As of September 2020, partnerships were developing around half of all COVID-19 vaccine candidates, including those in clinical trials. Almost half of those partnerships involved two research entities, and about 40 percent included a research entity and a player in the development, manufacturing, and/or commercialization spaces (Chagar et al., 2021). Inevitably, some of these partnerships will ebb post-pandemic, but others will likely facilitate more rapid access to vaccines. Moreover, effective partnerships should—in theory—become easier to form. As new products are developed, this could also contribute to expediting access to vaccines. For example, Indonesia serves as the regional hub for the production and distribution of Chinese vaccines across Southeast Asia (Nugroho, 2020).

In some cases, the crucible of the COVID-19 pandemic catalyzed an "all-hands-on-deck" attitude among traditional competitors in the pharmaceutical industry. For instance, Sanofi has partnered or plans to partner with the manufacturers of three major COVID-19 vaccines to expand production capacity. In January 2021, it announced plans to share access to its manufacturing infrastructure and expertise with Germany's BioNTech to produce 125 million vaccine doses, followed the next month by declaring a similar partnership with Johnson & Johnson to produce 12 million doses of its vaccine per month. Beginning in September 2021, Sanofi will partner with Moderna by using its manufacturing capacity and infrastructure to support the production of 200 million vaccine doses (Keown, 2021).

THE CURRENT STATE OF INFLUENZA VACCINE MANUFACTURING AND THE LIMITATIONS OF EGG-BASED VACCINES

If the COVID-19 pandemic had been caused by influenza, it is unclear whether vaccine access would have been broader. Three types of seasonal influenza vaccines are available: (1) inactivated influenza vaccines (IIVs), (2) live attenuated influenza vaccines (LAIVs), and (3) recombinant vaccines. Both IIVs and LAIVs can be manufactured using embryonated chicken eggs as the substrate; IIVs can also rely on an animal cell–based substrate that does not require chicken eggs. In contrast, recombinant vaccines are manufactured synthetically without requiring a candidate vaccine virus (CVV) sample. The substrate for production of these vaccines is either egg based (i.e., using embryonated chicken eggs) or cell based (using cell culture).

In 2019, the 12-month global production capacity for seasonal and pandemic influenza was estimated to be 1.48 billion doses for the former if manufacturers were operating at full-scale capacity (Sparrow et al., 2021) and for the latter, 4.15 billion doses assuming "moderate case" production capacity and 8.31 billion doses for "best-case" capacity. The global production of all influenza vaccines remains highly reliant on egg-based processes: in 2019, egg- and cell-based vaccines represented 84.5 percent and 15.5 percent, respectively, of the global production capacity for seasonal vaccines. Of the overall pandemic influenza vaccine production capacity, 79 percent was egg based and 21 percent cell based.[2] The vast majority of global production capacity is used for IIVs (seasonal: 89.6 percent; pandemic: 88.9 percent), followed by recombinant vaccines (seasonal: 5.4 percent; pandemic: 7.7 percent) and LAIVs (seasonal: 5.0 percent; pandemic: 3.4 percent).

Influenza vaccines are manufactured using a distributed model, although the majority of the production capacity—particularly for pandemic influenza—is located in high-income countries (HICs). According to the analysis of global production capacity of seasonal and pandemic influenza vaccines in 2019 (Sparrow et al., 2021), the distribution of the 40 active production facilities by World Health Organization (WHO) region is skewed toward the Western Pacific Region (20 facilities), although active facilities were located in all regions except for the African Region (European Region: 9; Region of the Americas: 7; South-East Asia Region: 3; Eastern Mediterranean Region: 1) (Sparrow et al., 2021). None was located in low-income countries, while 20 facilities were in HICs, representing 69 percent of global seasonal vaccine production capacity and 80 percent of pandemic vaccine production capacity. Of the remaining 20 facilities, 15 were located in upper-middle-income countries and five in low- and middle-income countries (LMICs).

[2] These proportions are different from those for seasonal vaccine production because two manufacturers who produce seasonal vaccines in eggs have approval to produce cell-based vaccines for pandemics, some of the manufacturers with cell-based productions produce quadrivalent vaccines, and one manufacturer has an approved facility for cell-based IIV for a pandemic but does not produce seasonal flu vaccines.

Existing production facilities for seasonal influenza could be switched over to produce pandemic influenza vaccines. However, even in the best-case scenario, it would take 4–6 months after the declaration of a pandemic for vaccines to be available for deployment and months longer to maximize production capacity (Sparrow et al., 2021). For an entirely new IIV, it would take at least 23–24 weeks after selecting the virus and uploading its genetic sequence to produce the first doses.[3] LAIVs have a slightly shorter time from sequencing to deployment, about 21 weeks. Recombinant vaccines can be produced on a much more rapid time line than either, largely because they are not dependent on a CVV, but they represent only a small fraction of the current global vaccine production capacity.

The technologies that dominate the influenza vaccine manufacturing system are, therefore, not optimal. While egg-based technologies have a long history and an excellent safety profile, they have limited efficacy (ranging from 60 percent in 2010–2011 to only 10 percent in 2004–2005) (NASEM, 2019), longer production times, and susceptibility to bottlenecks in the production process. Manufacturing capacity could be expanded using cell culture (i.e., producing antigens), but this has even lower yields than eggs (although some new technologies, such as strain modification, may allow cell culture to produce higher yields). Recombinant technologies have shown high productivity for influenza but would also lead to shortages of adjuvants.

The mRNA and platform technologies could potentially manufacture vaccines more rapidly than the egg-based method, which could also contribute to containing and controlling the spread of influenza. However, the egg-dominated market might have deterred some manufacturers from taking the risk on mRNA and other new technologies if the world had been hit by an influenza pandemic instead. On the other hand, an influenza pandemic could also have given mRNA and other recombinant technologies an earlier proving ground than COVID-19, and some companies might have attempted to apply mRNA or other new platforms to influenza. Successes with new platforms could relatively quickly render egg-based technology obsolete.

NEW TECHNOLOGIES FOR INFLUENZA ON THE HORIZON

Such new technologies are on the horizon for influenza but still far from ready for widespread rollout. In recent years, the field of influenza vaccine platform technology has expanded significantly, with 106 vaccine

---

[3] Timing includes the time needed for (1) the CVV to be prepared, characterized, safety tested by the reassorting laboratories, and shipped to manufacturers; (2) the manufacturers to assess the CVVs for yield and growth characteristics, prepare clinical lots, and conduct clinical trials and for vaccine production, formulation, packaging, and distribution; (3) the Essential Regulatory Laboratories to prepare reagents necessary to measure potency and for lot release; and (4) national regulatory authorities to assess the vaccine for licensure and release it.

candidates in various clinical trial phases. As of July 2021, 26 new technologies had reached clinical trials, and 90 were in the late preclinical trial stage, according to the Universal Influenza Vaccine Technology Landscape (CIDRAP, 2021). Figure 4-2 provides a visual depiction of the global vaccine landscape at the preclinical and early clinical trial phases, with six different types of platforms: recombinant proteins, non-virus-like particles (nanoparticles), virus-like particles (VLPs), virus-vectored, nucleic acid, and recombinant influenza virus. Table 4-2 provides a breakdown of the vaccine platforms by clinical trial phase, with a significant number (85 out of 106) in the preclinical phase.

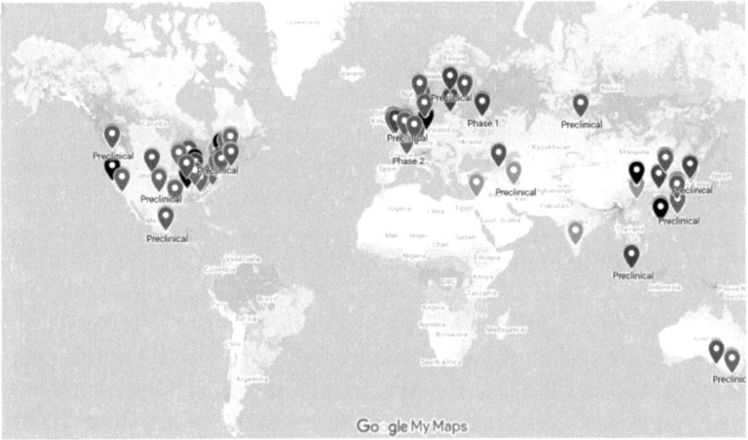

FIGURE 4-2 Broad visual depiction of the global influenza vaccine development platform landscape.
SOURCE: Based on data from CIDRAP (2021), as of June 1, 2021. https://ivr.cidrap.umn.edu (accessed December 19, 2021).

TABLE 4-2 Influenza Vaccine Platforms by Clinical Trial Phase

	Vaccine Platform						
Clinical Trial Phase	Recombinant Proteins	Non-Virus-Like Nano-particles	Virus-Like Particles	Virus Vectored	Nucleic Acid Based	Recombinant Influenza Virus Based	**Total**
Preclinical	19	17	16	13	13	7	85
Phase I	3	2	1	1	2	2	11
Phase II	1	1	0	3	0	2	7
Phase III	1	1	1	0	0	0	3
Total	24	21	18	17	15	11	**106**

SOURCE: Data from CIDRAP (2021), as of June 1, 2021. https://ivr.cidrap.umn.edu (accessed December 19, 2021).

Recombinant Technology Vaccines

Recombinant technology vaccines in development for influenza include quadrivalent vaccines, VLPs, and nanoparticles. Quadrivalent technology (FluBlok, Sanofi Pasteur, Lyon) involves using genetically modified baculoviruses to insert tailored RNA into insect cells, where vaccine proteins are then grown. Initial research suggests that the FluBlock vaccine may be at least 30 percent more efficacious than the standard vaccines in adults aged >50 years (Venkatesen, 2017). VLPs (Medicago, Quebec) are used to produce recombinant DNA VLP vaccines in tobacco leaf cells (Ward et al., 2021) and could allow for vaccine production to begin just 5–6 weeks after the declaration of a pandemic if the virus strain is known. As of 2019, this technology was in Phase III trials. Nanoparticle technology being developed by Novavax showed a favorable safety profile, which was confirmed in Phase III trials.[4]

mRNA Vaccines

As of May 2019, Phase I clinical trials had tested two first-generation mRNA vaccines (Moderna, Norwood MA) against two highly pathogenic influenza strains (Bender, 2019). In 2018, Pfizer and BioNTech announced a partnership to develop mRNA influenza vaccine, with BioNTech to receive $120 million up front from Pfizer plus up to $305 million more, depending on development achievement; tiered royalties on future sales were expected to be in the double-digit percentage range (Reuters, 2018). In January 2021, Moderna announced three new vaccine programs targeting seasonal influenza, HIV, and Nipah virus. The company also expects to extend mRNA work to 24 programs in five therapeutic areas. The influenza vaccines—mRNA-1010, mRNA-1020, and mRNA-1030—will target seasonal types A and B (Laguipo, 2021). In April 2021, Moderna's chief executive officer, Stephane Bancel, announced that it is planning to develop an influenza vaccine in tandem with its COVID vaccine as a single booster shot (Bever, 2021).

ACCELERATING THE DEVELOPMENT OF PLATFORM TECHNOLOGIES FOR INFLUENZA

Accelerating the development of platform technologies for influenza vaccines over the next 3–5 years will enhance the speed of production and potential efficacy. While developing pre-pandemic strain-specific vaccines is viewed as an insurance policy, this approach is costly and may be futile if vaccines for a putative pandemic strain are never needed because the pandemic does not materialize, as happened with the 2005 H5N1 influenza

---

[4] See https://www.novavax.com/our-pipeline#nanoflu (accessed December 19, 2021).

outbreak. Viruses also have time to mutate over the required 6 months or more needed for egg-based technologies, which compromises the efficacy of the final product, as occurred with the H7N9 vaccine in 2017. Post hoc development of vaccines has also often been an ineffective response to a pandemic given the slowness of egg-based technologies.

A universal influenza vaccine would represent a real game changer and eliminate or greatly reduce all of these problems at once. Progress is under way on multiple fronts—from R&D to financing—to develop this holy grail. Ideally, it would confer 3–5 years of protection from morbidity and mortality caused by all influenza A subtype viruses and influenza B lineage viruses, both circulating and emerging ("drifted and shifted"). The 2018 Strategic Plan developed by NIH's National Institute of Allergy and Infectious Diseases (NIAID) highlights NIAID's commitment to support the research needed to advance the development of a universal influenza vaccine that provides long-lasting protection against multiple strains for both seasonal and potentially pandemic influenza (Erbelding et al., 2018). The European Union's Framework Programme for Research and Technological Development, part of Horizon 2020, also supports major initiatives to develop novel influenza vaccines through (1) improving understanding of immunity against the virus and immune response to vaccines; (2) identifying genetic biomarkers that characterize highly pathogenic strains; and (3) using new immunization technologies, formulations, and vectors and delivery systems, and vaccination methods (Navarro-Torné et al., 2019). The European Union expects that its Joint Influenza Vaccine Effectiveness Studies program will positively influence societal acceptance of influenza vaccines in Europe, result in improved vaccine coverage, and ultimately reduce the burden of disease. If it proves a successful model, it could be expanded to other vaccines in EU national and subnational immunization programs.

Development of a universal influenza vaccine is garnering financial support from various philanthropic donors and initiatives. In 2018, the Bill & Melinda Gates Foundation (BMGF) partnered with FluLab to launch a $12 million Universal Influenza Vaccine Development Grand Challenge seeking bold, innovative, and transformative ideas to be realized through interdisciplinary collaboration outside of the scope of traditional efforts. In the same year, the Wellcome Trust announced its support for the Center for Infectious Disease Research and Policy (CIDRAP) to develop a roadmap for R&D for influenza vaccines to accelerate progress toward universal or broadly protective influenza vaccines; it was published in September 2021.[5]

A 2020 report by the Sabin-Aspen Vaccine Science and Policy Group surveyed the current state of progress toward a universal influenza vaccine,

[5] See https://www.cidrap.umn.edu/ongoing-programs/influenza-vaccines-roadmap (accessed December 19, 2021).

noting that the rate of research, development, and innovation has generally decelerated in recent years, despite substantial investments in basic research. It will likely remain stagnant if the vaccine market remains focused and reliant on outdated processes for tracking and selecting likely seasonal virus strains and using egg-based manufacturing processes, both of which deter investment and innovation toward a universal vaccine. The group argued that accelerating development will require overcoming the fragmentation and lack of goal-oriented coordination that pervades the system by (1) creating an entity to lead and coordinate this effort, (2) advancing an R&D agenda focused on transformational change that includes a broader range of scientific perspectives, and (3) communicating the true impact of influenza and the urgent need for a universal vaccine.

A number of entities could play such a role in a universal vaccine effort if their mandates and missions were expanded. For example, CEPI is a global partnership among public, private, philanthropic, and civil society organizations; its mission[6] is to "accelerate the development of vaccines against emerging infectious diseases and enable equitable access to these vaccines for people during outbreaks."[7] CEPI has identified a number of gaps in the landscape that it was designed to fill. First, CEPI works to counter known threats through "proof-of-concept safety testing" and will establish vaccine stockpiles as a preparedness measure. Second, CEPI funds new and innovative platform technologies with a potential to "accelerate the development and manufacturing of vaccines against unknown pathogens," with an intent to meet a time line of 16 weeks from antigen identification to product release for clinical trials. Third, CEPI supports and coordinates activities to improve the collective response to epidemics, strengthen capacity in at-risk countries, and advance the regulatory science that governs vaccine development. CEPI has no *specific* role in the influenza ecosystem, but an expanded mandate could allow it to lead a global effort for developing a universal influenza vaccine if supported by sufficient funding.

Another entity that could play a leading or coordinating role in the search for a universal influenza vaccine is BARDA.[8] It prepares for the next influenza pandemic by supporting development, licensure, and manufacturing of improved products to detect, treat, and prevent seasonal and pandemic influenza, which can be rapidly manufactured. BARDA has a strong track record of bringing medical countermeasures for influenza across the finish line, supporting a broad portfolio of pandemic countermeasures licensed or approved by the U.S. Food and Drug Administration. By

---

[6] See https://cepi.net/about/whyweexist (accessed December 19, 2021).
[7] See https://cepi.net (accessed December 19, 2021).
[8] See https://www.phe.gov/about/barda/Pages/PI.aspx (accessed December 19, 2021).

partnering with industry product developers and manufacturers, BARDA supports developing cutting-edge influenza vaccines, diagnostics, and therapeutics and maintains stockpiles of influenza vaccine antigens and adjuvants. However, it is a U.S. government agency and not charged with global international coordination as its major focus.

In February 2021, the European Commission (EC) announced a proposal for its Health Emergency Preparedness and Response Authority (HERA) Incubator, premised on the understanding that expanding vaccine production capacity in Europe would require more integrated and strategic public–private partnerships with the pharmaceutical industry. The EC also established the Task Force for Industrial Scale-Up of COVID-19 Vaccines to help ramp up production capacity and alleviate supply chain bottlenecks (Hoen et al., 2021). HERA is currently primarily focused on variants of SARS-CoV-2 that are causing great concern because of their increased transmissibility. The European Union is setting up a European biodefense preparedness plan "HERA Incubator" to bring together researchers, biotech companies, manufacturers, regulators, and public authorities to monitor variants, exchange data, and cooperate on adapting vaccines. The plan will focus on detecting, analyzing, and adapting to virus variants; speeding up regulatory approval of vaccines; providing guidance on data requirements and facilitating the certification of new or repurposed manufacturing infrastructures; and supporting the speedy mass production of adapted or novel COVID-19 vaccines. The EU investment in state-of-the-art vaccine and drug R&D and manufacturing capacities will be one of the core blocks for future pandemic response but will also contribute to EU strategic autonomy in the area of health and the positioning of the European health care industry. It is, however, just being organized at the time of this report.

Other entities might be able to play a role in coordinating and leading a push for a universal influenza vaccine. The Global Funders Consortium for Universal Influenza Vaccine Development, established in 2017 to convene organizations and governments that fund R&D for universal influenza vaccines in particular, has been and can continue to be involved in identifying funding gaps and promoting dialogue between key stakeholders.

It is the committee's consensus that CEPI merits serious consideration for wider global coordination. Its current mission and mandate, including its investment case emphasis on developing a universal vaccine against coronaviruses, would allow it to assume this role. This would not require an extensive mission expansion but would benefit from expanding CEPI's support of "platform-agnostic" technologies. It will also be important to improve coordination for future influenza vaccine research at CEPI and/or HERA and BARDA with institutional R&D capabilities that go beyond the United States, particularly in Germany (e.g., Max Planck Institutes), Japan, and South Korea, and engage regional entities for R&D mobilization.

While the remarkable effectiveness of mRNA vaccines against SAR-CoV-2 makes the technology attractive for many vaccines, a universal influenza vaccine is still a science problem more than a manufacturing problem. Toggling between seasonal and pandemic influenza vaccine production has long been considered the best strategy to maintain a "warm" base for a pandemic vaccine when it is needed, and platform technologies offer an opportunity to move beyond this dynamic because they could be used for seasonal influenza vaccines and other pathogens.

GEOGRAPHICALLY DISTRIBUTED AND REGIONAL MANUFACTURING MODELS ("HUBS")

Momentum is gathering toward a shift to models such as distributed manufacturing and regional development hubs that bring vaccine production closer to the end users. Greater scale in global manufacturing capacity could reduce the extent of rationing in a pandemic; greater geographic distribution of global manufacturing capacity could reduce the inequalities of access that arise in rationing. However, a trade-off exists between these two approaches.

For influenza and other types of vaccines using new platform technologies, this shift could help drive much broader and more equitable access worldwide. This momentum is reflected in the G20 Summit's 2021 Rome Declaration, which calls for voluntary licensing and technology transfer to increase global production of COVID-19 vaccines and has spurred billions of dollars in pledges from G20 members and vaccine manufacturers (Talor, 2021). At the same summit, the EC announced that it will provide €1 billion in support for a Team Europe initiative on manufacturing and access to vaccines, medicines, and health technologies in Africa (European Commission, 2021).

In a pandemic, LMICs that do not have local vaccine production capacity or contractual supply agreements with producers of medical countermeasures must rely on internationally coordinated pandemic influenza vaccine deployment. Sustainable local manufacturing capacity is one way to address the risk of inequitable and delayed vaccine availability (WHO, 2013). In June 2021, The Rockefeller Foundation urged G7 leaders to adopt its Updated Action Plan for Global COVID-19 Vaccination, which calls for regional manufacturing hubs in the Global South to narrow the gap between vaccine manufacturing capacity between the developed and developing worlds (The Rockefeller Foundation, 2021).

The aim of decentralized manufacturing is to reduce delays and gaps in access to vaccines through regional production. The basic premise of "decentralized" or "distributed" manufacturing is that it disperses production across various locations (Harrison et al., 2018). Adopting this model alters manufacturers' organizational structure in a range of advantageous ways, such as democratizing supply, creating additional jobs in more locations, and allowing more flexibility in response to changes in demand. Distributed supply chain hubs in parallel to manufacturing facilities also present a market opportunity for countries to supply the bags, filters, and other items required for vaccine supply chains. This model differs from the "hub-and-spoke model," whereby vaccines can be stored in ultra-cold freezers in centralized production "hubs" and then transported to regional "spokes" for short-term storage and administration, because decentralized facilities are not reliant on a central manufacturing hub.

However, decentralization also raises challenges related to ensuring oversight, unified decision making, stressing the supply chain, maintaining product quality, and ensuring a downstream market (demand for the products). None of these are specific to influenza vaccine production. No global institutional architecture exists to handle them, and development finance institutions often struggle to establish business cases for developing vaccines for a pandemic event with uncertain timing. During COVID-19, CEPI performed early manufacturing scale-up, and BARDA-supported scale-up through Operation Warp Speed (OWS), but this support was provided *after* the pandemic began. In addition, any expansion in production capacity must be accompanied by expanding suppliers of raw materials and consumables, which presents another set of challenges.

The argument for the regional hub model is particularly strong in Africa, which had received less than 2 percent of COVID-19 vaccines worldwide as of April 2021 (WHO, 2021). In April 2021, WHO issued a global call for "expression of interest" in establishing COVID-19 mRNA vaccine technology transfer hubs, which could scale up production and access. Through a partnership with COVAX, the Africa Centres for Disease Control and Prevention (CDC), a network of universities, and an industry consortium (Biovac, Afrigen Biologics and Vaccines), the first such hub is planned for South Africa. This is a crucial step in building geographically distributed manufacturing hub capacity, but additional investments will be necessary on a much larger scale. Between April and June 2021, the Partnership for Africa Vaccine Manufacturing was also launched by the Africa CDC and the African Union. The goal of the partnership is that by 2040, African countries should produce at least 60 percent of the vaccines they use, as opposed to the current 1 percent (Africa CDC and African Union, 2021). In April 2021, Rwandan president Paul Kagame also remarked that Rwanda has also discussed creating an mRNA vaccine plant.

One potential manufacturer, GreenLight BioSciences, has proposed small, modular mRNA plants that can be built in Massachusetts and shipped worldwide. Each could take advantage of its own locally sourced raw materials and potentially provide up to 17 million doses per month at an estimated cost of about $200 million per mini-vaccine plant (Greenlight, 2021). Similar momentum is building in the Latin America and Caribbean regions. As of May 2021, only 3 percent of the population in Latin American countries were fully vaccinated for COVID-19, leading Pan American Health Organization (PAHO) Director Christine Etienne to call for regional hub development: "We must ramp up production for the entire vaccine value chain—from the ingredients that go into vaccines to the vials and syringes that help us deliver them—without compromising quality" (PAHO, 2021).

Geographically distributed manufacturing is a largely unregulated field. Regional manufacturers have struggled to know what others are working on and where they may obtain relevant technical advice and training, which must be kept up to date for quality, safety, and efficiency. CEPI recently (May 2021) launched a survey[9] to map the landscape of vaccine manufacturing capacity and capability in Africa, Southeast Asia, the Middle East, and Latin America. These issues will also need to be addressed to facilitate establishing effective and successful regional hubs. Political and economic stability, and other factors related to regulatory, infrastructural, and supply chain capacity, must be part of the equation for planning future geographically distributed manufacturing hubs, if they are to be effective and sustainable.

CAPABILITIES REQUIRED FOR THE TRANSITION TO PLATFORM TECHNOLOGIES

An inevitable consequence of the shift from egg-based vaccines to platform technologies will be a transitional period of several years for seasonal vaccine manufacturing characterized by a degree of instability and uncertainty. To support the transition and increase influenza vaccine production capacity, six capabilities are required, all of which rely on strong global partnerships:

1. **Robust early-phase R&D**—particularly Phase III clinical trials—focused on platform technologies for influenza and, ideally, a platform-based universal influenza vaccine;
2. Sufficient worldwide **capacity for manufacturing vaccines** to facilitate the success of distributed or regional hubs;
3. Effective **business models** to drive demand and use facilities for products other than pandemic vaccines;
4. **Systematic workforce training** for sustainable technology transfer and a nimble response to subsequent shifts in technologies;
5. Expansion of regionally integrated **regulatory capacity** for vaccines; and
6. Appropriate consideration of end users' needs and **supply chain** bottlenecks, particularly for a geographically distributed hub model.

---

[9] See https://cepi.net/news_cepi/survey-launched-by-cepi-to-track-multinational-vaccine-manufacturing-capacity-for-use-in-future-epidemics-and-pandemics (accessed December 19, 2021).

BARRIERS AND PATHWAYS TO SUCCESS FOR EFFECTIVE GLOBAL PARTNERSHIPS TO SUPPORT NEXT-GENERATION INFLUENZA VACCINES

This section surveys current barriers and pathways to success for effective global partnerships for influenza vaccine development and manufacturing based on each of these essential capabilities for influenza vaccine production.

R&D: Barriers

The unprecedented pace of vaccine R&D propelled by the COVID-19 pandemic demonstrated the value that can be achieved through cooperation and resource pooling. However, it also exposed a range of "orphan problems" in the development landscape, which no entity is accountable for addressing in a pandemic context (Sabin-Aspen Vaccine Science and Policy Group, 2021), including the lack of mechanisms for (1) sharing newly discovered viral strains and subsequent mutations, (2) safeguarding intellectual property rights, (3) ensuring liability protection, and (4) harmonizing regulatory processes. It also highlighted the need for advance planning to forge partnerships to rapidly develop and test new vaccines in LMICs.

The gaps identified in CIDRAP's Influenza Vaccines Research and Development Roadmap mirror many of these wider orphan problems and barriers in the domains of policy, governance, financing, and regulation (Moore et al., 2021). For instance, substantial financing risks and inadequate incentives are significant barriers to bringing broadly protective vaccines to market (WHO, 2016). The "valley of death" refers to the phases spanning early discovery, to Phase III clinical trials, to regulatory approval and early commercialization, when manufacturers bear a disproportionate and asymmetrical burden of the risk. For example, they incur substantial R&D and licensure costs, despite uncertain or risky outcomes and no revenue yet generated or guaranteed. This can be a substantial disincentive to enter the vaccine market (Douglas and Samant, 2018). Barriers also inhibit the later phases—Phase III trials, licensure, and monitoring—that require the greatest financial inputs but lack global coordination and sustainable, collaborative models with appropriate market incentives (Rappuoli et al., 2021). Gaps in R&D governance include no coordinated commitment to funding R&D for universal influenza vaccines, which warrants new public–private partnerships similar to those established for COVID-19 vaccine development (Krammer et al., 2018).

The predominant commercial model for global vaccine production is based on annual reformulation and egg-based technology, which is a barrier to investing in new vaccines with a potentially broader effect. This underscores the need to consider innovative strategies for financing the development of new types of influenza vaccines (Douglas and Samant, 2018). Improving vaccine effectiveness, coupled with more attractive "branding" through coordinated communications strategies, could help to stimulate investment in innovative R&D strategies. Developing innovative approaches will require substantial additional investments in infrastructure across R&D and production—particularly to overcome challenges during the valley of death. Coordinated partnerships involving national governments, the pharmaceutical industry, philanthropic organizations, and academia will be critical in advancing new vaccines through clinical trials and licensure (Bresee et al., 2019). As Nicole Lurie has recommended, "For future outbreaks and potential pandemics, it is crucial to identify key areas of research as quickly as possible, and have established mechanisms to rapidly release funds from a pre-positioned pool to jumpstart the research and development response" (Lurie et al., 2021, p. 1234).

Further barriers are posed by a lack of transparent sharing of technology information that would allow scientists worldwide to collaborate on innovations (Kavanagh et al., 2021). For instance, the platform designed by the Global Research Collaboration for Infectious Disease Preparedness (GloPID-R) supports scientists and research funders in identifying optimal research solutions and channeling the necessary funds into those solutions rapidly, which also conserves resources and avoids duplication. Glopid-R has facilitated collaboration between India and the European Union focused on next-generation influenza vaccines (Chaudhury, 2020). However, its role is limited to coordination and information sharing among research funders. Moreover, although it includes 29 major research funders, it lacks sufficient financial backing. Although GloPID-R is a valuable first step, such platforms must be supported by sufficient mandates and resources to be significantly impactful (Lurie et al., 2021).

The Ebola vaccine is a cautionary example of failure to adequately coordinate R&D across public–private partnerships; poor coordination delayed deployment of an existing vaccine until 1 year into the epidemic. In addition to the absence of shared protocols, global authorities did not clearly communicate how many doses would be needed. The vaccine candidate that ultimately proved effective (VSV-ZEBOV; now licensed as Ervebo) had been developed a decade earlier and could have been advanced and ready to deploy much sooner given appropriate pathways and incentives (Sabin-Aspen Vaccine Science and Policy Group, 2021).

R&D: Partnership Pathways for Success

Elements from OWS offer instructive examples of how partnerships can help forge pathways for success in vaccine R&D. For instance, OWS facilitated the selection of multiple platforms and companies, then provided coordinated assistance to companies at multiple steps along the development chain. Specifically, the partnership between the U.S. Department of Defense (DoD) and the U.S. Department of Health and Human Services (HHS) spurred the quickest vaccine development in history by providing at-risk funding for manufacturing and testing candidates from five companies—AstraZeneca, Janssen Pharmaceuticals (a unit of Johnson & Johnson), Moderna Inc., Novavax Inc., and Sanofi. (Pfizer Inc. opted to use its own resources for its COVID-19 vaccine.) Although OWS was successful in accelerating the development of safe and effective vaccines, it was less successful in expanding manufacturing capacity and facilitating the administration of those vaccines, with around 2–3-fold fewer vaccine doses administered than planned.

A major boon to OWS was the use of clear criteria for company selection based on robust preclinical and early-stage clinical trial data that suggested the potential to enter Phase III field efficacy trials between July and November 2020, with outcomes by the first half of 2021. Additional criteria included platform technologies permitting rapid, effective manufacturing and companies that demonstrated industrial process scalability, yields, and consistency such that they would be capable of producing more than 100 million doses by mid-2021. Moreover, OWS selected different platforms to mitigate the risk that any single platform or specific vaccine candidate would fail due to any number of problems related to safety, efficacy, industrial manufacturability, and scheduling. OWS included two platforms that had not been used in a licensed vaccine but theoretically could be quickly adapted and scaled up (the mRNA and replication-defective live-vector platforms) and one that had been proven—the recombinant-subunit-adjuvanted protein platform.

The approaches adopted by OWS also enabled customized partnerships with each pharmaceutical company, thus allowing for tailored support of all major aspects of the vaccine development chain. For instance, Pfizer was provided with a financial incentive to bear the R&D risk. The other five companies were required to adhere to published "tenets" as a condition of receiving support. For those companies, OWS took on 80–100 percent of the financial risk by funding both R&D and manufacturing. If Phase III trials had failed, all funding would have been provided by the U.S. government. Furthermore NIH network–associated clinical trial sites—representing 20–40 percent of sites—were engaged to operationalize the Phase I–III trials. Although Pfizer manufactured its own vaccine, OWS was involved in all operational aspects of manufacturing for Moderna's vaccine, including accessing and ordering raw materials, obtaining special equipment and machinery, installation, and other support. The other four companies used sites for drug substance manufacturing that were part of a BARDA collaborative network. Alongside technical teams from those companies, OWS supported the equipping of sites, hiring of talent, and validating of work to support scale-up of manufacturing (GAO, 2021).

Markets and Business Models: Barriers for Pandemic Flu Vaccines

The Sabin-Aspen Vaccine Science and Policy Group identified two major barriers to effective vaccine markets that are not specific, but are applicable, to influenza vaccines. The first is the misalignment between financial incentives and public health needs (the "profit-based model"); the second is the disproportionate concentration of markets in HICs.

About 80 percent of the US$ value of the global vaccine market is generated in HICs, despite those countries accounting for roughly only 20 percent of the annual volume of vaccines consumed (Shulman et al. 2021). LMICs account for about 18 percent of the dollar value of the global vaccine market but approximately 80 percent of the annual volume (WHO, 2019a). Manufacturers deeply entrenched in the influenza vaccine market have a residual commitment to arguing that a separate capacity needs to be retained for seasonal influenza. The complexity of the manufacturing process generally requires building new plants for each vaccine—which can take up to 5 years at a cost of at least $350 million in the United States or $150 million in India (Sabin-Aspen Vaccine Science and Policy Group, 2021). Concerns also abound regarding the fate of egg-based vaccine production facilities worldwide when companies with next-generation mRNA technologies begin to apply them to influenza vaccines.

A delicate balance must be struck between having facilities keep capacity warm between pandemics without relying on them absolutely for routine production. Although this issue will persist with the advent of new technologies, diversification could contribute to greater efficiencies (Sell et al., 2021). Either manufacturing capacity will need to be rapidly rolled out but not always needed or billions of dollars will need to be spent building capacities that are unnecessary in steady-state situations and cannot transition to necessary products. It is clear that the latter option is probably infeasible. Additional concerns proliferate around how to maintain trained staff and current regulatory licenses to enable rapid activation in a pandemic. From the manufacturers' perspective, however, it is impracticable to operate at 10 percent capacity to prepare for ramping up to 100 percent in an emergency. Mechanisms for initiating the switch after WHO declares a Public Health Emergency of International Concern (PHEIC) are still not agreed upon and often remain at the discretion of individual countries (Rockman et al., 2020). From the manufacturers' standpoint, switching means taking on major risk and potentially losing the return on a huge investment.

The WHO Global Action Plan (GAP) manufacturing program (2006–2019) was designed to bolster the market for influenza vaccines and sustainably increase manufacturing capacity. GAP aimed to increase the supply of a pandemic vaccine and thereby reduce the gap between the potential vaccine demand and supply anticipated during an influenza pandemic (WHO, n.d.).[10] The GAP experience offers three valuable lessons (see Box 4-1): (1) the development and manufacture of influenza vaccines is highly complex,

---

[10] See https://www.who.int/influenza_vaccines_plan/resources/gap_faq.pdf?ua=1 (accessed December 19, 2021).

BOX 4-1
Lessons Learned from the Global Action Plan for Influenza Vaccines (GAP) Influenza Manufacturing Capacity-Building Partnerships

Countries are notably different in their abilities to respond to a global influenza pandemic. The Global Action Plan for Influenza Vaccines (GAP) was born from a consultation organized by the World Health Organization (WHO) in May 2006. Representatives from national immunization programs, national regulatory authorities, vaccine manufacturers, and the research community met to develop plans for the long-term objective of vaccinating 70 percent of the global population. GAP identified the strengthening of seasonal influenza vaccine programs as a key measure toward improving pandemic influenza vaccine coverage. GAP proposed three primary goals: increasing (1) seasonal vaccine programs as a driver of increased market and production, (2) vaccine production capabilities, and 3) influenza vaccine research and development (Bright, 2012).

In partnership with the Biomedical Advanced Research and Development Authority (BARDA) and PATH, GAP launched a manufacturing capacity-building and technology transfer project. This project, which ran from 2006 to 2019, made seed funding and technical support available to vaccine manufacturers in low- and middle-income countries (LMICs) interested in influenza (Grohmann et al., 2016). This partnership was integral to GAP's successes. BARDA brought key resources to the collaboration, including access to technical and subject-matter experts and established relationships with multinational pharmaceutical companies, international government organizations, and nongovernmental organizations. Support from GAP and BARDA generated backing from government entities and manufacturers; investments from local manufacturers ultimately amounted to approximately 17 times that of the GAP/BARDA investment (BARDA, n.d.).

WHO created a Technical Advisory Group (TAG) to review grants submitted by manufacturers from LMICs interested in developing influenza vaccine production capacity. TAG members were also responsible for conducting site visits and reviewing grantees' quarterly reports. Access to this type of expertise was invaluable, as most of the grant recipients had never produced influenza vaccines before (Francis and Grohmann, 2011). Fourteen grantees received funding from GAP/BARDA, totaling $50 million. Countries receiving grants were Brazil, China, Egypt, India, Indonesia, Islamic Republic of Iran, Kazakhstan, Mexico, Republic of Korea, Romania, Serbia, South Africa, Thailand, and Vietnam.

At the conclusion of the program, successful grantees (those with a licensed vaccine and current functional facility) were capable of producing approximately 675.2 million doses of influenza vaccines within 12 months. In the project period (2006–2019), China, Vietnam, India, South Korea, and Brazil developed pandemic flu vaccine capacity. Since the program ended, additional gains have been made. In 2020, Torak in Serbia received licensing for a vaccine, and the Thai Government Pharmaceutical Organization (GPO) will likely have a sustainable vaccine licensed in 2022. Bio Farma, an Indonesian manufacturer, received financial support from the Indonesian government and signed an agreement with Biken Institute in Japan to cover the transfer of technology. While Bio Farma has reported progress toward its goals, at the time of writing, it had not succeeded in increasing production capacity

(Suhardono et al., 2011). After recent successful clinical trials, the Research Institute for Biological Safety Problems in Kazakhstan has secured national funding to build a full-scale production facility. In Romania, after previously having its vaccine banned by the National Agency for Medicines and Medical Devices because of endotoxin contamination, Cantacuzio is working to re-establish vaccine capacity. In Mexico, Birmex has moved into the fill and finish phase with Sanofi.

Among GAP/BARDA grantees, only manufacturers in Iran, Egypt, and South Africa have been unsuccessful at building their influenza vaccine capacity. Over the course of the wider GAP program (2006–2019), seasonal influenza vaccine production capability increased from 500 million to 1.47 billion doses and pandemic vaccine production capacity increased from approximately 1.5 to 6.37 billion doses (McLean et al., 2016). GAP grantees comprehensively therefore represent about 8.13 percent of the global pandemic production capacity. While the overall enhanced capacity among grantees marks a major success, participating LMICs still only produced a small fraction of the global capacity when the program ended in May 2019. In addition to increasing production capacity, grantees and funders held workshops and meetings, strengthening international partnerships and improving communication and information-sharing.

Pathways to Success:

1. **Commitment from national governments:** Manufacturers that were eager to participate nevertheless had to receive official support from a ministerial agency before they could receive funding and begin training or production. This political buy-in, particularly when it led to their own investments, proved crucial. Overall, governments and companies provided $1 billion compared with the WHO investment of $50 million (Grohmann et al., 2016). Some governmental bodies embraced program goals and provided supplemental funding. In Thailand, for instance, progress was initially slow due to political instability, but the program was ultimately successful, with the government investing $40–$50 million in building a full-scale production facility. Thailand is currently doing necessary clinical trials to be approved for production at industrial scale (Sparrow et al., 2021). Similarly, in Brazil, Anvisa's commitment to purchasing products from Instituto Butantan has made the program highly successful. In contrast, Egypt and the manufacturer Vacsera struggled due to limited political buy-in and the lack of a local market for vaccines produced (Sparrow et al., 2021).
2. **Sustained workforce training:** Developing a skilled workforce at each participating manufacturing facility was essential. Ideally, countries came into the program with at least general knowledge of vaccine manufacturing production capability, such as quality control/quality assurance and fill-finish operations. Successes of the program were in large part due to sustained injections of "know-how" from BARDA subject-matter experts, the TAG, and PATH consultants. Critically, this included experts with regulatory, industry, and vaccine R&D skills. There were two pathways for workforce development. One was based on sending manufacturing staff to two facilities in the United States for hands-on training, with the

continued

BOX 4-1 Continued

goal of developing a workforce network of vaccine manufacturers from LMICs. Manufacturers nominated 2–3 people each year for this training. The second pathway, supported by PATH and BARDA, was hands-on training in a manufacturer's own facilities (Sparrow et al., 2021). These two pathways were supplemented by a technology hub in the Netherlands and an annual meeting among grant recipients to provide updates and share experiences. Together, these strategies led to beneficial collaborations between LMIC manufacturers, such as a knowledge exchange between China and the Serum Institute of India, and led to training more than 250 technical staff from LMICs (BARDA, n.d.).

3. **National regulatory functionality:** For a vaccine to be produced and distributed in any country or region, manufacturers must receive approval from the local regulatory authority. The functionality of that authority and/or reliance agreements with WHO or other countries is therefore essential for vaccines produced to be brought quickly to market. The program recognized this fact and had parallel projects to develop regulatory capacity with WHO and the U.S. Food and Drug Administration (FDA). Workforce development activities also lead to assistance with the design of clinical trial protocols, which are essential for licensure (Sparrow et al., 2021).
4. **Early consideration of market demand:** One of the most common failure points for GAP program grantees was related to a lack

for both egg-based vaccines and forthcoming novel-platform technologies; (2) the parallel time lines for manufacturing and developing demand for vaccines are interdependent and both equivalently years long; and (3) it is critical to think deeply about creating demand, especially if the technology has narrow applications. GAP leadership indicates that, if launching a similar initiative now, they would likely look beyond both the egg-based and "seasonal influenza vaccine market" models.

Markets and Business Models: Pathway to Success

Few blueprints exist for how to keep facilities warm, although mRNA technologies could transform this landscape (WHO, 2013). However, to address these challenges, a wealth of resources and expertise can be provided by regional and global industrial organizations, such as the African Vaccine Manufacturing Initiative, Developing Country Vaccine Manufacturing Network (DCVMN), Developing Country Vaccine Regulatory Network, Association of South-East Asian Nations, and International Federation of Pharmaceutical Manufacturers & Associations (WHO, 2013). Organizations of market demand for seasonal vaccines. When the program was conceived in 2005, WHO viewed egg-based seasonal influenza vaccine manufacturing as the best way to keep pandemic vaccine production "warm." A few years into the program, there was a push for sustainability assessments in countries, in which Ministries of Trade, Finance, and Health—as well as other stakeholders—were brought to the table to consider how to sustain local markets. This did not provide a resolution to all market issues, but did help countries to improve their decisions about vaccine absorptive capacity and the need for realistic national planning. In Serbia, for instance, the Torlak Institute received regulatory approval for a seasonal influenza vaccine last year, and it has been in discussions with WHO about options for sustaining its market, particularly given the quadrivalent vaccines available in Europe (Sparrow et al., 2021).

5. **Long-term commitment from all stakeholders:** The program reinforced that simply throwing money into manufacturing in LMICs will not build capacity without sufficient time. WHO underscores that strategic thinking about markets and national capacity required 5–10 years or more of buy-in, from WHO, grantees, and technical partners. For instance, having a multi-year commitment for the BARDA/PATH workforce training proved to be very valuable; the first year, manufacturers mostly sent senior people, while subsequent years allowed a more junior "back bench" to be trained (Sparrow et al., 2021).

such as the DCVMN, which are supported through public–private partnerships or foundations, have successfully expanded capacity to meet demand in certain regions—especially in parts of Latin America (Sabin-Aspen Vaccine Science and Policy Group, 2021). Gavi and BMGF investments have helped to counter incentives that drive production of high-margin vaccines, contributing to an increase in the number of companies producing basic vaccines for low-income countries (from 5 in 2000 to 18 in 2020) (Sabin-Aspen Vaccine Science and Policy Group, 2021). It will be critical to encourage greater involvement of coordination structures, such as the DCVMN. Unlike multinationals, participating countries rely heavily on grants, loans, and seed funding from public and philanthropic sources. For instance, at least half the non-influenza-specific vaccine doses procured by Gavi and UNICEF in recent years have come through the DCVMN (Hayman and Pagliusi, 2020).

Manufacturing Capacity: Barriers

In the push for distributed manufacturing, it is important not to underestimate the difficulties intrinsic to actually accomplishing one-time technology transfers. Simplistic distributed manufacturing initiatives may not be appropriate or successful (WHO, 2011). An analysis by the MIT Center for Biomedical Innovation of distributed versus centralized biologics manufacturing identified areas of cost efficiencies (MIT Center for Biomedical Innovation, 2017). Figure 4-3 summarizes the scenario: a centralized model with a single high-volume plant is replaced by six smaller, distributed plants with the same total production capacity. The cost centers in this model were qualitatively ranked as being better (strength/green in Figure 4-3), approximately the same (similar/yellow), or worse (weakness/red); while the model indicates that distributed production can provide efficiencies (such as the time to product access), it is also predicts critical increases in operational and regulatory costs.

Attempts to promote distributed manufacturing of antiretrovirals have not been widely successful. A critical factor for success (or failure) of these efforts is the commitment from LMIC governments. Major barriers encountered are the need for steady and consistent government policy, adequate infrastructure, qualified technical and managerial human resources, robust production-distribution logistics systems, strong national regulatory agencies, and an international market (Pinheiro Edos et al., 2014).

GAP (2006–2019) and BARDA's International Influenza Vaccine Manufacturing Capacity Building Program employed a partnership model based on distributed, egg-based vaccine manufacturing capacity (see Box 4-1). GAP was supported by an independent technical advisory group (Francis and

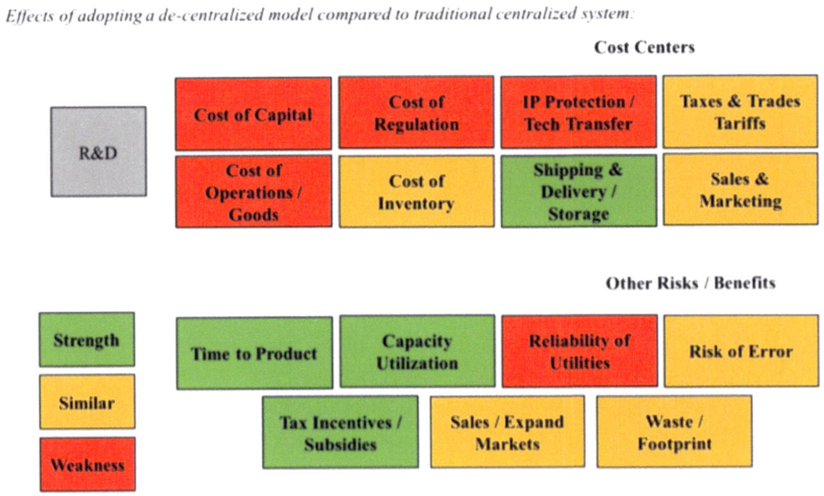

FIGURE 4-3 Expected change in cost centers and other non-cost variables when comparing a centralized model with a decentralized system, each producing the same total product volume.
SOURCE: MIT Center for Biomedical Innovation, 2017.

Grohmann, 2018) to assist WHO in selecting proposals for funding and providing programmatic support for successful grantees. Participation in this voluntary program was based on manufacturers' submitting letters of intent to WHO declaring their interest in developing influenza pandemic vaccine capacity. Across the program's lifetime, 14 manufacturers were provided with financial support over four review processes (2007, 2009, 2011, 2013); WHO allocated approximately $50 million through 2015. According to BARDA, every $1 of funding leveraged $17 in local investment. Despite the program's successes, it was merely a drop in the bucket in terms of expanding global vaccine manufacturing capacity. It was estimated that successful grantees with a licensed vaccine and functional facility could collectively produce a maximum of 675.2 million doses of pandemic vaccine in 12 months, which represented only 8.13 percent of the total global capacity in 2019.

Manufacturing Capacity: Partnership Pathways to Success

As illustrated by the GAP program, distributed vaccine production has many pathways to failure and a narrow road to success (McLean et al., 2016). It is critical to consider both the distributed manufacturing location and capacity. For instance, small-scale country manufacturing could be sufficient to meet a country's own needs, whereas larger capacity operations in countries with small populations could allow for rapid production to support regional needs. As demonstrated by the cooperation among PATH, BARDA, and GAP, multi-agency involvement can leverage agencies' respective strengths—for example, BARDA financed PATH's involvement, particularly in the arena of workforce development.

Lessons learned from GAP suggest the following key predictors of success for a program aiming to expand manufacturing capacity through partnerships (see Box 4-1):

1. Political will and stability, which can be bolstered by requiring all manufacturers applying to a program to send a letter of support from their ministerial agency;
2. Large-scale investment from local governments;
3. A skilled workforce, even if it is only experienced with basic vaccine quality assurance, quality control, and fill-finishing;
4. A strong regulatory agency, with involvement of WHO/U.S. Food and Drug Administration (FDA) regulatory systems and training opportunities; and
5. Available expertise for in-facility training, such as subject-matter experts, technical advisory groups (including ex-industry and regulatory expertise), or a pool of consultants.

OWS underscored the importance of providing coordination and assistance to companies about how to form partnerships to address limited manufacturing capacity. For example, BARDA assisted one company in identifying an additional manufacturing partner to increase production, and the U.S. Army Corps of Engineers oversaw construction projects to expand capacity at vaccine facilities. The Partnership for Influenza Vaccine Introduction (PIVI) further highlighted the value and necessity of long-term sustained investment in generating demand.

Various models can be implemented to apply these predictors of success to future programs, ranging from distributed models, to picking some "winners" for continued capacity (i.e., geographically distributed hubs), to manufacturer trade-offs in wealthy countries. With a fully distributed model, it is not possible to achieve the economies of scale needed to attain low-cost manufacturing. According to an analysis of scale of production and its influence on costs for influenza vaccines at WHO, manufacturing costs were much greater at a small than a large scale. Although local production might seem like the best option for achieving a sustainable supply, governments may not have considered how this strategy may increase costs. Decisions about engaging in country-based distributed manufacturing should be underpinned by national buy-in and a full understanding that vaccines may be more expensive.

Workforce Development and Technology Transfer: Barriers

In terms of driving manufacturing to capacity, human capital is often more important than monetary capital. The worldwide dearth of experts who have experience with critical technology and quality control processes presents a substantial challenge for distributed manufacturing. No global facilities or consortia exist to train personnel for full-scale vaccine R&D and manufacturing or connect stakeholders across all elements of the time line (Cawein et al., 2017). Additionally, a larger trained workforce is necessary to assist funders, such as the World Bank, in assessing and monitoring projects. Barriers to workforce development include the requirements for both sustained investment and high-level country buy-in over the long term, which is challenging in the face of changing political and organizational and administrations.

Workforce Development and Technology Transfer: Pathways to Success

GAP had a dedicated focus on workforce development, which was a key element of its success. Both Utah State University and North Carolina State University provided hands-on training to the program's workforce, which included support in clinical development and the design of clinical trial protocols. At BARDA-supported academic institutions, more than 250 technical staff from developing countries attended vaccine manufacturing training programs coupled with onsite technical support. BARDA also partnered with PATH to provide targeted technical support to manufacturers of influenza vaccines nearing eligibility for licensure.

The GAP experience illustrates that training over a few years is critical: manufacturers were encouraged to send 2–3 staff members to these facilities each year, which was reinforced with onsite training. Over several years, this contributed to building a "back bench." Another valuable workforce development strategy is an annual meeting onsite as a forum for providing updates and sharing experiences. For example, SII engaged in knowledge exchange with China while building its LAIV manufacturing capacity. Similarly, assistance in addressing workforce gaps was a critical component of OWS's success in increasing yields; DoD collaborated to expedite visa approval for key technical personnel, including technicians and engineers needed to assist with installing, testing, and certifying critical equipment from overseas. DoD personnel were also requested to serve as quality control staff at two manufacturing sites.

Regulatory Capacity: Barriers

Obtaining regulatory approval for vaccines requires national regulators to be experienced in assessing and monitoring sites for compliance with core Good Manufacturing Practice principles, especially for new sites. However, some LMICs lack sufficient capacity to provide rapid expert reviews of novel vaccines and thus rely on evaluations by agencies in other countries. This contributes to delays in licensing (and therefore access), lack of harmonized standards for ensuring product safety, efficacy, and quality, and problems with labeling and packaging. It also often leads to inconsistent local, and additional clinical trial, requirements (Sabin-Aspen Vaccine Science Policy Group, 2021).

In many LMICs, this limited or absent regulatory capacity is linked to the lack of national seasonal influenza vaccine policies. An evaluation of such policies in 194 WHO member states from 2014 to 2018 was conducted through the WHO/UNICEF Joint Reporting Form on Immunization to chart the evolution of influenza pandemic preparedness and identify challenges in sustaining equitable vaccine access (Morales et al., 2021). In 2018, only 79 percent (154 countries) reported influenza data via the form; 103 consistently had vaccination policies, and 65 consistently provided no evidence of a policy. Policies were most frequent in the WHO Regions of the Americas (89 percent of countries) and Europe (89 percent); they were less frequent in the Western Pacific (62 percent), Eastern Mediterranean (57 percent), Southeast Asia (27 percent), and Africa (11 percent). The type of vaccine technology used was not widely known, especially in low-income countries (WHO, 2019b).

Regulatory Capacity: Partnership Pathways to Success

It can be difficult for vaccine manufacturers to navigate the regulatory pathway of establishing the superiority of their technology through appropriate efficacy markers. This is a particular challenge for geographically distributed hub models. Partnerships forged during the COVID-19 pandemic have demonstrated WHO's crucial role. It coordinates vaccine approvals internationally through its Prequalification Program, established in 2001, and also employs its Emergency Use Listing procedure for vaccines. WHO can help enable swift authorization of products for use in countries with limited ability to conduct their own evaluations (Sabin-Aspen Vaccine Science and Policy Group, 2021).

The Africa CDC Consortium for COVID-19 Vaccine Clinical Trials, launched July 2020 by the African Union Commission, may provide an instructive example of how to regionally support testing, regulatory approval, and access to COVID-19 vaccines in alignment with geographically distributed hubs (Africa CDC, 2020). Developing the Ebola vaccine also illustrates the benefits of providing prequalification and early regulatory guidance for vaccines in LMICs. Designating the Ebola vaccine as a breakthrough therapy with priority review status triggered a fast-track mechanism that allowed FDA to provide intensive guidance at the earliest phases of clinical trials. As part of the review process, FDA coordinated with international regulatory agencies and based its approval, in part, on research conducted outside of the United States (Fritz, 2020; Sabin-Aspen Vaccine Science Policy Group, 2021).

Supply Chain Partnerships: Barriers

A substantial barrier in the vaccine supply chain is lack of coordination with end users about their health systems' capacity to absorb vaccines and ancillary supplies during a pandemic. During the COVID-19 pandemic, input supply challenges were observed across all steps in the vaccine manufacturing process, including bioreactor bags, single-use systems, cell-culture media, filters, upstream and downstream gamma sterilization, and fill-and-finish supplies, such as vials. Such individual challenges are amplified via compounded risk, whereby the absence of any single input can disturb the entire process. This is linked to the limited data available for forecasting supplies and manufacturing needs, which requires collaboration between public and private sectors followed by clear communication of the potential forecasted needs (IFPMA, 2021). Multinational organizations are often reluctant to rapidly adopt single-use systems due to concerns that specific supplies may not be available. Thus, strategies to approach and strengthen the connectivity of single-use systems warrant careful consideration.

Supply Chain Partnerships: Pathways to Success

An effective supply chain requires three components: (1) interchangeability (developing a "USB style"), (2) diversification to manage redundancy, and (3) speed and flexibility from regulators. The transition to mRNA vaccines and platform technologies requires highly specialized equipment and personnel. In addition to the need for sufficient available capacity (e.g., trained workforce to perform quality control), the input supply chain is critically important. This includes raw materials, consumables, and equipment across the value chain (i.e., upstream, downstream, and through to fill-and-finish). Some of these inputs are common to all types of vaccines and even to other biologic therapeutics; however, other inputs are specific to each technology platform. Certain materials, such as glass vials, are associated with significant risks in the upstream supply chain (IFPMA, 2021).

Lessons learned during the COVID-19 pandemic reveal many opportunities to reinforce supply chains. It highlighted the critical importance of developing multidisciplinary, government, and expert-led partnerships with the ability to build and commandeer lists of critical supplies, in order to avoid supply chain breakdowns, coordinate their delivery, and prioritize contracts. OWS provided federal assistance to address manufacturing supply chain challenges. This contribution effectively facilitated manufacturing COVID-19 vaccines when—due to global demand—companies were waiting 4–12 weeks for items that would have been available for shipment in about 1 week pre-pandemic. Through the program, DoD and HHS provided federal assistance to (1) expedite procurement and delivery of critical manufacturing equipment, (2) develop lists of critical supplies common across the six OWS vaccine candidates, (3) expedite delivery of necessary equipment and goods to the United States, and (4) place prioritized ratings on 18 supply contracts for vaccine companies under the Defense Production Act.

The UK Vaccine Task Force, launched in May 2020, included experts from the military and pharmaceutical industry and civil servants with expertise in preclinical and clinical development, regulatory issues, manufacturing, and project management. Close support by the UK government in building supply chains for pharmaceutical firms, and "effectively commandeering" a manufacturing facility while securing exclusive access to another, have been cited as major factors in the success of this effort (Hoen et al., 2021).

KEY FINDINGS AND CONCLUSIONS

Fostering Influenza Platform Innovation

- The current vaccine manufacturing capacity for influenza vaccines would be insufficient to vaccinate the world, even over 12 months.
- The goal in the next 3–5 years should be to progressively pursue development and assessment of new platform technologies to improve vaccine effectiveness and expand the technology options to optimize vaccine production. A universal influenza vaccine could be a game changer that could take the threat of influenza—both seasonal and pandemic—off the table. Platform innovation will require a combination of early R&D incentives, including support of Phase I–III clinical trials for platform and recombinant-based technologies.
- Encouraging and incentivizing *voluntary* industry partnerships will assist with developing platform technologies—and initiating their technology transfer—and should also be designed to support the partnerships needed for a universal influenza and/or next-generation vaccines. Because of the competitive nature of the vaccine enterprise, this sharing should take place under the auspices of government partnerships, with appropriate intellectual property protections.
- Several existing organizations may be able to lead large-scale R&D and clinical trials for influenza platform technologies, including large-scale global action in LMICs, if they are given expanded mandates that are matched with significant infusions of funding. These could include CEPI, BARDA, and the HERA Incubator.
- As a public–private partnership with a multilateral approach, CEPI has an existing platform with scientific expertise and networks that span the first three steps in the vaccine development process: preclinical development, clinical development, and scale-up (Yamey et al., 2020). Adding funding for the advanced development could provide transaction cost efficiency compared to launching a new mechanism, and large investments could allow CEPI to extend its expertise to Phase III trials and potentially technology transfer.
- OWS is another example of what might work for influenza vaccine platform development, both for R&D and for manufacturing scalability to have surge capacity during a pandemic. The approach employed by OWS for COVID-19 vaccines was to support a variety of technologies, recognizing that the most effective platform for a particular antigenic target in a newly emerged pathogen will remain unknown until later phases of development. OWS provided

federal assistance to address supply chain challenges, which effectively facilitated manufacturing by reducing waiting times during a period of high demand. Federal assistance was also provided to expedite both procuring and delivering critical manufacturing equipment and delivering necessary equipment and goods to the United States. Other program attributes include its strong central management, sufficient funding for its objectives, and high level of oversight. Giving BARDA a broader remit may allow it to overcome one limitation of OWS: it did not account for global need by building out how the United States works with industry.

- It will be important to improve coordination for future influenza vaccine research at CEPI, HERA, BARDA, and NIAID; build institutional R&D capabilities beyond the United States, such as in Germany (e.g., Max Planck Institute), Japan, and South Korea; and engage regional entities for R&D mobilization.

Supporting Geographically Distributed Regional Manufacturing Hubs

- Geographically distributed manufacturing hubs are a way to provide scaled-up vaccine manufacturing in LMICs. The difficulty is in how to scale up industry partnerships and apply them globally, in support of a geographically distributed manufacturing hub model.
- Sustainable and successful geographically distributed manufacturing hubs face several challenges in the context of influenza vaccination. They require (1) government commitment and strong industry involvement, (2) strong business models, (3) the capacity to develop a product that can be licensed and exported (e.g., workforce training for technology transfer and regulatory capacity), and (4) keeping national plans updated, to guide who will get vaccines, where, and how.
- The GAP program focused on egg-based technologies; any future global partnerships for diversified manufacturing and supply chain coordination should be designed to sustain newer technologies and provide long-term demand certainties. Increasing seasonal influenza vaccine demand as a principle for expanding global manufacturing capacity will not be sufficient to generate a pandemic vaccine market on the scale required.
- Moving to geographically distributed manufacturing hubs requires significant inputs to ensure that the surrounding "ecosystem" is in place for technology transfer and workforce development for platform technologies, regulatory capacity to produce vaccines, and a business model that creates a market for products developed

using platform technologies (with the ability to rapidly switch to pandemic production mode) during times of no disease pandemics.

- A business model for pandemic influenza vaccines requires a dual-use paradigm for manufacturing facilities to keep them functioning between pandemics. This should encourage investment in platform technologies for vaccines for *both* seasonal influenza and other pathogens. It should pay at least as much attention to workforce development, regulation, and supply chain production as to manufacturing scale-up.
- This downstream market issue (demand for products developed) is different from upstream technology and R&D issues and not specific to influenza. No global institutional architecture exists to handle this issue, and development finance institutions often struggle to develop business cases for developing vaccines for a future pandemic event with uncertain timing.
- During COVID-19, supply chains broke down and have often been the reason that we could not produce more vaccines faster. Geographical distribution is not just about having factories and research facilities; it is also about ensuring that these factories have key inputs that they need to produce vaccines and the flexibility to diversify their production. Supply chain commodity production requires similar attributes.
- Developing geographically distributed supply chain hubs in parallel to manufacturing facilities presents a market opportunity for countries to invest as suppliers in the bags, filters, and other items required for vaccines. Supply chains are often treated as if they are only something you need for manufacturing, but being a supplier is also a business.

REFERENCES

Africa CDC (Centres for Disease Control and Prevention). 2020. *Africa CDC Consortium for COVID-19 vaccine clinical trials*. https://au.int/sites/default/files/documents/39350-doc-africa_cdc_consortium_for_COVID-19_clinical_trials_-_eng.pdf (accessed October 23, 2021).

Africa CDC and African Union. 2021. *Partnerships for African Vaccine Manufacturing (PAVM) Task Force communiqué: Africa projects 60% vaccines production by 2040*. https://www.thisdaylive.com/index.php/2021/06/29/africa-projects-60-vaccines-production-by-2040 (accessed December 30, 2021).

BARDA (Biomedical Advanced Research and Development Authority). n.d. *International influenza vaccine manufacturing capacity building program*. https://www.medicalcountermeasures.gov/barda/influenza-and-emerging-infectious-diseases/international-influenza-vaccine-manufacturing-capacity-building-program/ (accessed January 7, 2022).

Bender, E. 2019. Accelerating flu protection: Can the latest techniques speed up the dangerously slow production of flu vaccines? *Nature* 573:S60–S61. https://www.nature.com/articles/d41586-019-02756-5?error=cookies_not_supportedpercentcode=0d3fa8fb-ff26-49a4-8f74-2114493b6b6f (accessed July 22, 2021).

Bever, L. 2021. Coronavirus vaccine technology is paving the way for a whole new approach to flu shots. *The Washington Post*, April 11, 2021. Washington, DC.

Bresee, J. S., K. E. Lafond, M. McCarron, E. Azziz-Baumgartner, S. Y. Chu, M. Ebama, A. R. Hinman, A. Xeuatvongsa, S. Bino, D. Richardson, R. M. Porter, A. Moen, M. McKinlay, G. Sahakyan, S. Wangchuk, P. Ruowen, Z. Yongchao, C. Linlin, C. Daouda, O. Tarkhan-Mouravi, P. Gould, P. Muthoka, G. O. Emukule, S. S. Chaves, M.-A. Widdowson, D. Otorbaeva, V. Khanthamaly, K. Stavridis, V. Mikic, N. Furtuna, D. Capmari, B. Alexander, E. Dueger, M. Kamolzoda, J. Mott, A. Bin Salah, M. Mazur, A. Maria Ropero Alvarez, S. J. Olsen, S. Mirza, C. Sofia Arriola, J. Seward, S. Kluglein, A. F. Bolster, N. Minh Hang, J. W. McFarland, N. Ha Thu, and T. Thi Minh Nguyen. 2019. The partnership for influenza vaccine introduction (PIVI): Supporting influenza vaccine program development in low- and middle-income countries through public–private partnerships. *Vaccine* 37(35):5089–5095.

Cawein, A., E. Emini, M. Watson, J. Dailey, J. Donnelly, D. Tresnan, T. Evans, S. Plotkin, and W. Gruber. 2017. Human capital gaps in vaccine development: An issue for global vaccine development and global health. *Annals of the New York Academy of Sciences* 1395(1):3–11.

Chagar, A., M. Thomas, L. Zuo, and M. Watson. 2021. *The R&D response to COVID-19: What can we learn for the vaccine ecosystem?* Sabin-Aspen Vaccine Science and Policy Group. https://www.sabinaspengroup.org/the-rd-response-to-covid-19-what-can-we-learn-for-the-vaccine-ecosystem (accessed October 23, 2021).

Chaudhury, D. R. 2020. India, EU working to develop new generation of influenza vaccines: Envoy. *The Economic Times*. https://economictimes.indiatimes.com/industry/health care/biotech/health care/india-eu-working-to-develop-new-generation-of-influenza-vaccines-envoy/articleshow/75215403.cms?from=mdr (accessed December 19, 2021).

CIDRAP (Center for Infectious Disease Research and Policy). 2020. *Universal influenza vaccine technology landscape*. https://www.cidrap.umn.edu/universal-influenza-vaccine-technology-landscape (accessed July 20, 2021).

Douglas, R. G., and V. B. Samant. 2018. The vaccine industry. *Plotkin's Vaccines* 41–50.

Erbelding, E. J., D. J. Post, E. J. Stemmy, P. C. Roberts, A. D. Augustine, S. Ferguson, C. I. Paules, B. S. Graham, and A. S. Fauci. 2018. A universal influenza vaccine: The strategic plan for the National Institute of Allergy and Infectious Diseases. *The Journal of Infectious Diseases* 218(3):347–354.

European Commission. 2021. *1 billion Team Europe Initiative on manufacturing and access to vaccines, medicines and health technologies in Africa*. https://ec.europa.eu/commission/presscorner/detail/en/IP_21_2594 (accessed October 23, 2021).

Francis, D. P., and G. Grohmann. 2011. WHO Influenza Vaccine Technology Transfer Initiative: Role and activities of the Technical Advisory Group. *Vaccine* 29S:A45–A47.

Fritz, M. 2020. *Drug approval during a public health crisis*. Regulatory Review. https://www.theregreview.org/2020/02/11/fritz-drug-approval-during-public-health-crisis (accessed October 23, 2021).

GAO (U.S. Government Accountability Office). 2021. *Operation Warp Speed: Accelerated COVID-19 vaccine development status and efforts to address manufacturing challenges*. GAO-21-319. Washington, DC: U.S. Government Accountability Office.

Greenlight Biosciences. 2021. *A blueprint to vaccinate the world*. https://www.green light-biosciences.com/wp-content/uploads/2021/03/How-to-vaccinate-the-world-Green-Light-0326.pdf (accessed October 23, 2021).

Grohmann, G., D. P. Francis, J. Sokhey, and J. Robertson. 2016. Challenges and successes for the grantees and the Technical Advisory Group of WHO's influenza vaccine technology transfer initiative. *Vaccine* 34(45):5420–5424.

Harrison, R. P., S. Ruck, Q. A. Rafiq, and N. Medcalf. 2018. Decentralised manufacturing of cell and gene therapy products: Learning from other health care sectors. *Biotechnology Advances* 36(2):345–357.

Hayman, B., and S. Pagliusi. 2020. Emerging vaccine manufacturers are innovating for the next decade. *Vaccine X* 5:100066.

Hoen, E., C. Garrison, P. Boulet, K. Mara, and K. Perehudoff. 2021. *Scaling up vaccine production capacity: Legal challenges and recommendations.* Background paper 6. Commissioned by The Independent Panel for Pandemic Preparedness and Response. https://theindependentpanel.org/wp-content/uploads/2021/05/Background-paper-6-Scaling-up-vaccinationlegal-aspects.pdf (accessed October 24, 2021).

IFPMA (International Federation of Pharmaceutical Manufacturers & Associations). 2021. *Towards vaccinating the world: Landscape of current COVID-19 supply chain and manufacturing capacity, potential challenges, initial responses, and possible "solution space"—a discussion document.* https://www.ifpma.org/wp-content/uploads/2021/03/Summit_Landscape_Discussion_Document.pdf (accessed October 24, 2021).

Kavanaugh, M. M., L. O. Gostin, and M. Sunder. 2021. Sharing technology and vaccine doses to address global vaccine inequity and end the COVID-19 pandemic. *JAMA* 326(3):219–220.

Keown, A. 2021. *Sanofi partners with Moderna to answer global demand for COVID-19 vaccines.* https://www.biospace.com/article/sanofi-to-manufacture-200-million-doses-of-the-moderna-vaccine-its-third (accessed July 19, 2021).

Krammer, F., A. Garcia-Sastre, and P. Palese. 2018. Is it possible to develop a "universal" influenza virus vaccine?: Potential target antigens and critical aspects for a universal influenza vaccine. *Cold Spring Harbor Perspectives in Biology* 10(7):a028845.

Laguipo, A. 2021. *Moderna to develop three new mRNA-based vaccines against HIV, influenza, and the Nipah virus.* https://www.news-medical.net/news/20210113/Moderna-starts-to-develop-three-new-mRNA-based-vaccines-against-HIV-influenza-and-the-Nipah-virus.aspx (accessed October 23, 2021).

LaMattina, J. 2021. Beyond its COVID-19 vaccine, Pfizer's foray into flu vaccines can also prove lucrative. *Forbes,* May 6, 2021. https://www.forbes.com/sites/johnlamattina/2021/05/06/beyond-its-covid-19-vaccine-pfizers-foray-into-flu-vaccines-can-also-prove-lucrative/?sh=7794eac13306 (accessed July 19, 2021).

Lurie, N., G. T. Keusch, and V. J. Dzau. 2021. Urgent lessons from COVID-19: Why the world needs a standing, coordinated system and sustainable financing for global research and development. *The Lancet* 397(10280):1229–1236.

McLean, K. A., S. Goldin, C. Nannei, E. Sparrow, and G. Torelli. 2016. The 2015 global production capacity of seasonal and pandemic influenza vaccine. *Vaccine* 34(45):5410–5413.

MIT (Massachusetts Institute of Technology) Center for Biomedical Innovation. 2017. *Comparing centralized vs. distributed models of biologics manufacturing and supply for global health: A discussion of challenges and opportunities.* https://cbi.mit.edu/wp-content/uploads/2020/11/Scoping-Report-Global-Biologics-Supply.pdf (accessed July 21, 2021).

Moore, K., J. Ostrowsky, A. Kraigsley, A. Mehr, and M. Osterholm. 2021. *Commentary: From hope to reality: The promise of the influenza vaccines R&D roadmap.* https://www.cidrap.umn.edu/news-perspective/2021/01/commentary-hope-reality-promise-influenza-vaccines-rd-roadmap (accessed June 8, 2021).

Morales, K. F., D. W. Brown, L. Dumolard, C. Steulet, A. Vilajeliu, A. M. Ropero Alvarez, A. Moen, M. Friede, and P. Lambach. 2021. Seasonal influenza vaccination policies in the 194 WHO member states: The evolution of global influenza pandemic preparedness and the challenge of sustaining equitable vaccine access. *Vaccine* 8:100097.

NASEM (National Academies of Sciences, Engineering, and Medicine). 2019. *Exploring lessons learned from a century of outbreaks: Readiness for 2030: Proceedings of a workshop*. Washington, DC: The National Academies Press.

Navarro-Torné, A., F. Hanrahan, B. Kerstiëns, P. Aguar, and L. Matthiessen. 2019. Public health–driven research and innovation for next-generation influenza vaccines, European Union. *Emerging Infectious Diseases* 25(2):e180359.

Newland, M., D. Durham, J. Asher, J. J. Treanor, J. Seals, R. O. Donis, and R. A. Johnson. 2021. Improving pandemic preparedness through better, faster influenza vaccines. *Expert Review of Vaccines* 20(3):235–242.

Nugroho, A. 2020. *Indonesia is set to become the hub for Chinese vaccines in Southeast Asia. How does the country benefit?* https://theconversation.com/indonesia-is-set-to-become-the-hub-for-chinese-vaccines-in-southeast-asia-how-does-the-country-benefit-148534 (accessed October 24, 2021).

PAHO (Pan American Health Organization). 2021. *PAHO director calls for closing "glaring" vaccine gap by expanding vaccine production in Latin America and the Caribbean.* https://www.paho.org/en/news/19-5-2021-paho-director-calls-closing-glaring-vaccine-gap-expanding-vaccine-production-latin (accessed July 20, 2021).

Pinheiro Edos, S., K. Brüning, M. F. Macedo, and A. C. Siani. 2014. Production of antiretroviral drugs in middle- and low-income countries. *Antiviral Therapy* 19(Suppl 3):49–55.

Rappuoli, R., E. De Gregorio, G. Del Giudice, S. Phogat, S. Pecetta, M. Pizza, and E. Hanon. 2021. Vaccinology in the post–COVID-19 era. *Proceedings of the National Academy of Sciences* 118(3):e2020368118.

Reuters. 2018. *Pfizer bets on biotech flu vaccine in $425 million BioNTech alliance.* https://www.reuters.com/article/us-pfizer-biontech-alliance/pfizer-bets-on-biotech-flu-vaccine-in-425-million-biontech-alliance-idUSKBN1L10F5 (accessed July 20, 2021).

The Rockefeller Foundation. 2021. *One for all: An action plan for financing global vaccination and sustainable growth.* New York: The Rockefeller Foundation.

Rockman, S., K. Laurie, and I. Barr. 2020. Pandemic influenza vaccines: What did we learn from the 2009 pandemic and are we better prepared now? *Vaccines* 8(2):211.

Sabin-Aspen Vaccine Science and Policy Group. 2019. *Accelerating the development of a universal influenza vaccine.* https://www.aspeninstitute.org/wp-content/uploads/2019/07/sabin-aspen-report-digital.pdf (accessed July 20, 2021).

Sabin-Aspen Vaccine Science and Policy Group. 2021. *Powering vaccine R&D: Opportunities for transformation.* https://www.sabinaspengroup.org/powering-vaccine-rd-opportunities-for-transformation (accessed July 20, 2021).

Schafer, J., and Sparrow, E. 2021. *Lessons learned from the Global Action Plan for Influenza Vaccines (GAP)'s technology transfer partnerships and the Biomedical Advanced Research and Development Authority (BARDA)'s International Influenza Vaccine Technology Manufacturing Capacity Program.* https://www.nationalacademies.org/event/05-11-2021/lessons-learned-from-global-influenza-technology-transfer-partnerships-meeting-3-supplementary-session (accessed August 24, 2021).

Sell, T. K., D. Gastfriend, M. Watson, C. Watson, L. Richardson, L., A. Cicero, T. Inglesby, and N. Connell. 2021. Building the global vaccine manufacturing capacity needed to respond to pandemics. *Vaccine* 39(12):1667–1669.

Shulman, J., R. Ahsan, and K. O'Malley. 2021. *Understanding global vaccine economics and research and development.* Sabin-Aspen Vaccine Science and Policy Group. https://www.sabinaspengroup.org/understanding-global-vaccine-economics-and-research-and-development (accessed July 21, 2021).

Sparrow, E., J. G. Wood, C. Chadwick, A. T. Newall, S. Torvaldsen, A. Moen, and G. Torelli. 2021. Global production capacity of seasonal and pandemic influenza vaccines in 2019. *Vaccine* 39(3):512–520.

Talor, A. 2021. *The G20 pledge drive.* https://dukeghic.org/2021/05/25/the-g20-pledge-drive (accessed July 20, 2021).

Venkatesen, P. 2017. Recombinant influenza vaccine in adults aged 50 years or older. *The Lancet Respiratory Medicine* 5(8):613.

Ward, B. J., P. Gobeil, A. Séguin, J. Atkins, I. Boulay, P.-Y. Charbonneau, M. Couture, M-A. D'Aoust, J. Dhaliwall, C. Finkle, K. Hager, A. Mahmood, A. Makarkov, M. P. Cheng, S. Pillet, P. Schimke, S. St-Martin, S. Trépanier, and N. Landry. 2021. Phase 1 randomized trial of a plant-derived virus-like particle vaccine for COVID-19. *Natural Medicine* 27:1071–1078.

WHO (World Health Organization). 2011. *Increasing access to vaccines through technology transfer and local production.* Geneva, Switzerland: World Health Organization. https://www.who.int/phi/publications/Increasing_Access_to_Vaccines_Through_Technology_Transfer.pdf (accessed October 24, 2021).

WHO. 2013. *Report of the workshop on business modelling for sustainable influenza vaccine manufacturing.* Geneva, Switzerland: World Health Organization. https://www.who.int/influenza_vaccines_plan/resources/BusinessModeling_report_final.pdf (accessed December 19, 2021).

WHO. 2016. *Key elements of sustainability for influenza vaccine manufacturing in low- and middle-income countries.* Geneva, Switzerland: World Health Organization. https://apps.who.int/iris/bitstream/handle/10665/251695/WHO-HIS-TTi-GAP-16.3-eng.pdf?sequence=1isAllowed=y (accessed October 24, 2021).

WHO. 2019a. *Global vaccine market report.* Geneva, Switzerland: World Health Organization.

WHO. 2019b. *Partnership Contribution (PC) Preparedness High-Level Implementation Plan II 2018–2023, Revised Version.* Geneva, Switzerland: World Health Organization.

WHO. 2021. *WHO supporting South African consortium to establish first COVID mRNA vaccine technology transfer hub.* News Release, June 12, 2021. Geneva, Switzerland: World Health Organization. https://www.who.int/news/item/21-06-2021-WHO-supporting-South-African-consortium-to-establish-first-COVID-mRNA-vaccine-technology-transfer-hub (accessed October 24, 2021).

WHO. n.d. *Global Action Plan for Influenza Vaccines: Frequently asked questions.* https://www.who.int/influenza_vaccines_plan/resources/gap_faq.pdf?ua=1 (accessed December 19, 2021).

Yamey, G., M. Schäferhoff, M. Pate, M. Chawla, K. Ranson, F. Zhao, R. Hatchett, and R. Wilder. 2020. *Funding the development and manufacturing of COVID-19 vaccines. Duke* Global Working Paper 20. https://papers.ssrn.com/sol3/papers.cfm?abstract_id=3575660 (accessed December 17, 2021).

5

Influenza Vaccine Access and Financing

Despite new governance facilities aimed at promoting equitable access to COVID-19 vaccines—such as the COVID-19 Vaccines Global Access (COVAX) pillar of the Access to COVID-19 Tools (ACT) Accelerator—high-income countries (HICs) have cornered the market to the extent that major disparities in global access have emerged. In January 2021, the World Health Organization (WHO) Director-General Tedros Adhanom Ghebreyesus warned that in terms of ensuring access to COVID-19 vaccines, the world was "on the brink of a catastrophic moral failure—and the price of this failure will be paid with lives and livelihoods in the world's poorest countries" (WHO, 2021a). This mirrors the inequities that undercut access to vaccines during the 2009 H1N1 influenza pandemic (see Chapter 2). He echoed this sentiment in his opening remarks at the World Health Assembly (WHA) in May 2021, describing the ongoing vaccine crisis as a "scandalous inequity that is perpetuating the pandemic" (WHO, 2021b). Without improved coordination, incentivization, and investments to promote access in low-income countries (LICs), a similar pattern will likely undermine the rollout of vaccines during a future influenza pandemic.

THE COVAX FACILITY AND ITS SHORTFALLS

In April 2020, COVAX was formed jointly by WHO, the Coalition for Epidemic Preparedness Innovations (CEPI), and Gavi to invest in several vaccine candidates and ensure that the vaccines would be equitably distributed among participant countries largely by funding distribution to the 92 lowest-income countries. Box 5-1 provides an overview of its aims and financing structures. Almost every country signed up for COVAX, and it delivered its first doses in late February of 2021. The following month, due to the rapidly escalating number of cases in India, the Serum Institute of India (SII)—which COVAX had presumed would be its main vaccine supplier—stopped exporting its vaccine, which was made in collaboration with AstraZeneca and the University of Oxford (Cohen and Kupferschmidt, 2021). This move was predicted to create a 190-million dose shortage by the end of June 2021. COVAX had delivered just 4 percent of all vaccine doses administered worldwide as of May 2021, although its latest supply forecast (September 2021, WHO, 2021c) suggests that approximately 1.2 billion doses will be available for lower-income countries participating in its advance market commitment (AMC), enough to protect 40 percent of all adults in the 92 AMC countries, with the exception of India.

The COVAX experience highlights the difficulty facing global health coordination, particularly around broadening global access to vaccines in an era of geopolitical transformation and increasing nationalism. COVAX has certainly improved vaccine equity compared to a scenario without a multilateral procurement or allocation mechanism. However, progress toward equitable global vaccine allocation remains disappointing 18 months into the pandemic. The facility is unlikely to deliver doses representing 20 percent of each country's population by the end of 2021, as originally committed.

Ultimately, HICs mostly bypassed COVAX and pursued bilateral advance purchase; for instance, the United States and the European Union bought 3-fold more vaccines than they would need for their entire populations (Cohen and Kupferschmidt, 2021). Moreover, population coverage targets differed between self- and aid-financed countries. Figure 5-1 depicts the global share of individuals who received at least one dose as of mid-June 2021, starkly illustrating the extent to which the worldwide rollout has been inequitable for less wealthy nations.

Many of the challenges that fueled this disappointing COVAX performance operate out of its direct control. These include multiple forms of vaccine nationalism and associated lack of donor support and industry behavior. For instance, the time lost in coaxing HICs to join in 2020 contributed to delays in fundraising and resource mobilization, and heavy reliance on a few technologies and manufacturers (mostly based in the United States and the European Union) limited the speed and capacity of vaccine scale-up. It could be argued that the major "failure" of COVAX is naivety in anticipating these challenges. However, a more "anticipatory" design may not have made much difference in terms of access during a time of vaccine shortage and could have even had the unintended consequence of legitimizing the political economy of vaccine nationalism.

BOX 5-1
Overview of COVID-19 Vaccines Global Access (COVAX)

Objectives:

1. To create a global procurement mechanism to ensure equitable access to COVID-19 vaccines to all countries in the world.
2. To decide on the products and allocation of volume of doses for all the countries.
3. To give means to invest in research to ensure that vaccine development progressed as fast as possible.

Overall aims:

1. To drive down prices for all participants as a buyer with financial muscle.
2. To allocate vaccines at the same rate for both high-income countries and low- and middle-income countries, proportional to population size.
3. To be a lifeline for countries that have not entered any bilateral deals with vaccine manufacturers.

Financing structure:

1. Managed by Gavi, the Vaccine Alliance; Coalition for Epidemic Preparedness Innovations (CEPI); and World Health Organization (WHO)
2. Two-legged structure:
   a. *Self-financed:*
      - High-income countries, which would self-finance their own vaccines by paying upfront (by mid-September 2020).
      - A second category of purchase options called Optional Purchase Arrangement available to allow countries to opt in or out of certain products by requiring countries to pay higher proportion of total cost per dose upfront.
      - Population coverage target ceiling raised from 20 percent to 50 percent.

   b. *Aid-financed:*
      - 92 eligible low- and middle-income countries' vaccines would be financed completely by donor grant through an Advance Market Commitment.
      - Optional Purchase Arrangement not available.
      - Population coverage target: 20 percent.
3. US$8.3 billion for procurement and delivery of vaccines for 92 eligible low- and middle-income countries (as of June 2021).
4. Contractual obligation to provide one in five doses for high-income countries.

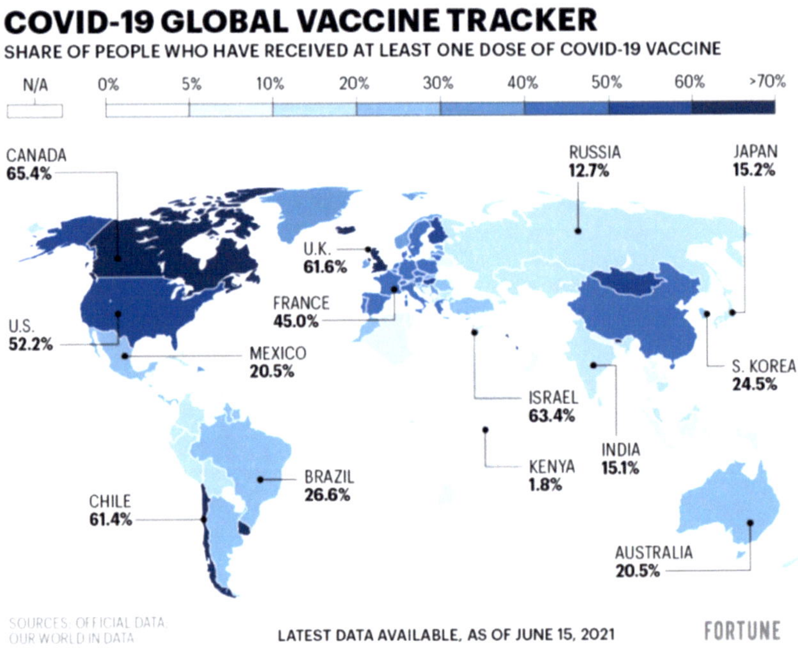

FIGURE 5-1 Global share of individuals who have received at least one dose of COVID-19 vaccine (as of June 15, 2021).
SOURCE: Our World in Data. https://bit.ly/3vdSoOv (accessed December 19, 2021).

The facility's self-finance window was perhaps a more avoidable design flaw. Inadequately self-financed HICs joined COVAX, which undermined its buying power. Most donor funds supplied through the AMC, which was used to finance the facility, were not pledged until late in the first half of 2021. Limited buying power had serious ramifications for inter- and intra-country equity in vaccine allocation and further limited the ability to support supply chains and manufacturing required for effective vaccine scale-up.

In response to this vaccine shortage and the vastly inequitable distribution of the limited supplies available, the "Financing Pandemic Preparedness and Response" paper commissioned by the Independent Panel for Pandemic Preparedness and Response (IPPPR), called on wealthy countries to donate 1 billion doses to COVAX by September 2021 and another 1 billion by the middle of 2022 (Radin and Eleftheriades, 2021). At the WHA, Ghebreyesus also called on all manufacturers to either offer any new product to COVAX before it enters the market or commit 50 percent of the doses to COVAX (Cohen and Kupferschmidt, 2021).

APPROACHING EQUITY IN VACCINE ACCESS FOR INFLUENZA

The COVID-19 pandemic has provided an unprecedented opportunity to move the needle on how equity is addressed in pandemic preparedness and response (PPR). Moral appeals can help to deal with equity issues during times of acute scarcities, but the reality is that policy makers need to be incentivized to promote equity. It is important to consider three questions when approaching issues of equity in access to influenza vaccines: (1) which strategies can be employed to improve equitable access, (2) what is the extent to which those strategies need to be specific to influenza, and (3) how much focus should be placed on equitable access to vaccines versus other medical products that are critical during a pandemic.

The question of how to improve equitable access spawns a set of further considerations related to whether equity should be dealt with directly or indirectly. It can be addressed directly either by considering equity and advancing discrete solutions—for example, via mechanisms such as WHO's Pandemic Influenza Preparedness (PIP) Framework—or through the physical location of production facilities (e.g., distributed manufacturing). Equity can be dealt with indirectly by increasing supplies to surge and building capacity to the degree that rationing becomes less biting. Michael Kremer of the University of Chicago has described the benefits equity principle, which holds that increasing supply naturally reduces the wait for everyone. Game theory shows that during a shortage, a gap emerges between social value and price; governments have powerful incentives to prioritize their domestic production, implement vaccine export bans, and hoard vaccines (Kremer, 2021). As a result, game theory predicts a lopsided vaccine allocation that prevents a socially (Pareto) optimal solution where global morbidity and mortality are reduced as much as possible. In practice, relying on principles of equity is not an effective tactic when scarcity is acute. Even when enshrined in law, equity access mechanisms are relatively ineffective during shortages. One strategy that can be useful during periods of acute scarcity is to ensure that capacity is in place with immediate inputs.

To the question of how specific to influenza the solutions to promote equitable access should be, Chapter 4 showed how the market for seasonal vaccination is limited to the extent that the basis may be insufficient to keep manufacturing warm for a pandemic. This is especially the case with the newfound potential transferability of platform technologies. If the focus is skewed toward the seasonal manufacturing base, the financing scale may be restricted to merely the tens of millions—not the hundreds of billions needed for a strong pandemic vaccine response.

How much focus should be placed on equitable access to vaccines during a pandemic versus other critical medical products is complicated by the mandate of the committee's Statement of Task (which is focused on vaccines and vaccination). However, vaccine financing solutions should not be siloed. When a new pandemic strikes, it is not possible to know a priori the optimal combination of containment measures, such as vaccines, diagnostics, and therapeutics. Ideally, coordination and financing mechanisms would have built-in flexibility to develop, manufacture, and deliver vaccines as well as other therapeutic tools.

LESSONS FROM THE COVID-19 VACCINE EXPERIENCE

At least three valuable lessons can be gleaned from COVID-19. First, paying up front to develop a portfolio of vaccine candidates and maintain sufficient surge manufacturing capacity can yield a huge return on investment. Second, having vaccine governance structures before a pandemic is essential. Third, such structures should specifically target how to achieve equitable access for low-income settings.

COVID-19 has demonstrated that it is critical to have vaccine governance structures and financing before a pandemic strikes, because it can alleviate the scarcity and perverse nationalism that underpin and exacerbate global inequities. Up-front financing is needed not only for manufacturing capacity but also to facilitate pre-procurement of vaccines and therapeutics prior to the lengthy process of obtaining full regulatory approval. The pandemic illustrated how paying for overcapacity to deliver vaccines during a pandemic is an inexpensive and cost-effective strategy. If there were a single decision-making entity for the world, it would likely maintain that spending several billion dollars per year on pandemic preparedness is highly rational. For example, Operation Warp Speed (OWS) paid for itself many times over: with a cost of $13 billion, it would have paid for itself in just 12 hours by virtue of accelerated vaccinations. Furthermore, the global benefits of the first 3 billion doses likely generated worldwide social benefits of $17.4 trillion, or $5,800 in benefits per course (Kremer, 2021).

Vaccine governance structures should specifically target low-income settings whose varied funding needs are often overlooked during a response, as seen during the COVID-19 pandemic. To work toward developing systems that promote access to vaccines against future pathogens with pandemic potential, the needs of low-income settings should be considered specifically, rather than looking at funding considerations from an exclusively global perspective. In this sense, reframing acceptable wait times for pandemic vaccines could be heralded as a major achievement of the COVID-19 pandemic response. The global dialogue now centers on whether the poorest countries can receive vaccines 2–3 months rather than 2–3 years after wealthier countries. This represents a seismic shift in what is regarded as acceptable access.

HOW HAS PANDEMIC FINANCING CHANGED DURING COVID-19?: FUNDING FOR COVID-19 PREPAREDNESS AND RESPONSE

In 2019, $374 million—representing less than 1 percent of overall official development assistance for health (DAH)—was spent on strengthening pandemic preparedness in low- and middle-income countries (LMICs) (Figure 5-2). Another $5.2 billion was spent on strengthening health systems, some of which could improve countries' ability to deal with epidemics and pandemics. However, even this volume of spending has been shrinking. Since 2003, global aid for health system strengthening has fallen from 22 to 14 percent of overall annual DAH (Burwell et al., 2020). Major mechanisms used to finance PPR at WHO, the World Bank, and other multilaterals include emergency/contingency funds, pandemic insurance bonds, pooled/block funding, and liability insurance (NASEM, 2016). Table 5-1 provides an overview of each category of financing modalities. However, these modalities are largely aimed at "response" rather than "preparedness." Preparedness spending is mainly a by-product of other health system spending. For example, Global Fund grants make significant contributions

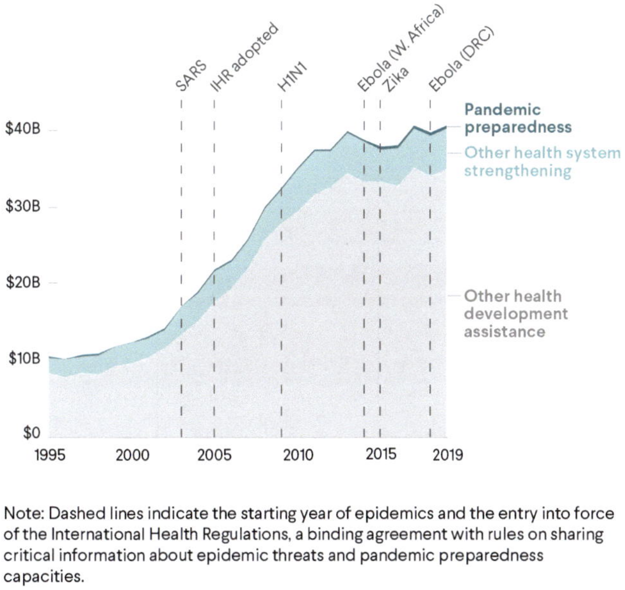

FIGURE 5-2 Global development assistance for health (2019 dollars).
SOURCE: https://www.cfr.org/report/pandemic-preparedness-lessons-COVID-19/pdf/TFR_Pandemic_Preparedness.pdf (accessed December 19, 2021).

TABLE 5-1 Types of Financing Modalities Used for Pandemics

Type of Financing Modality	Examples	Year of Inception	Overview	Level of Funding
Emergency/ contingency funds	WHO Contingency Fund for Emergencies (CFE)	2016	A rapidly available (24 hours or less), post-Ebola source of funding established by the UN General Assembly to respond to disease outbreaks and health emergencies (including natural disasters and armed conflict) but not earmarked for other health activities.	US$77 million (2018–2019)
	The UN Central Emergency Response Fund (CERF)	2006		US$35.8 million (2017) for the Democratic Republic of the Congo (DRC) during its Ebola outbreak
Pandemic insurance bonds for complex, contested risks	The World Bank Pandemic Emergency Financing (PEF) Facility	2017	A "catastrophe-bond" issuing system that offered additional opportunity for financial markets to diversify from traditional forms of investment (with a prospect of a return) to help the world's poorest countries respond to cross-border, large-scale outbreaks. This hit major hurdles, particularly its tight requirement for specific trigger criteria to be met, which is limited to seven viruses (including influenza) and requires cases to be confirmed in more than one country.	US$61.4 million for DRC to fight Ebola (including $50 million for the 10th outbreak)
	The African Risk Capacity (ARC) Outbreak and Epidemic Insurance Programme	Intended first issue of Cat bond or reinsurance cover in 2021	With funding from The Rockefeller Foundation and Swiss Agency for Development and Cooperation and strategic and technical support from the Africa Centres for Disease Control and Prevention and the WHO Regional Office for Africa, the ARC developed a sovereign parametric insurance product to address the financing needs of member countries to contain public health emergencies arising out of common infectious diseases in Africa.	Unknown

Pooled/block funding	*To be further developed:* An objective outbreak-focused integrated framework for disbursements	—	An integrated system that directs funds to responders from a central, impartial, coordinating body with exclusive remit to protect/improve global public health—best to be WHO. Actors would need to prove that they are worthy of investment. Donor preferences to fund particular activities should be incorporated into a WHO-led financial redistribution system targeting each outbreak when it occurs to appeal to the donors. Accompanied by a transparent system of accountability, effective use of technology, and strong leadership.	—
	Multilateral vaccine tiered-pricing system, the Global Alliance for Vaccines and Immunization (Gavi)	2000	A dynamic resource mobilization model to expand vaccines of hepatitis B (Hep B) monovalent, tetravalent (DTP3-Hep B), and pentavalent (DTP3-Hep B-Haemophilus influenzae type b); pneumococcal; and rotavirus. The model reaches out to current and new public and private partners with a diversified portfolio of instruments (direct contributions, innovative finance mechanisms and platforms), increases ownership of implementing countries through co-financing, influences market shaping through new market entrants and price reductions in vaccine manufacturing, and mobilizes advocacy of civil society networks while involving a wide range of partners.	US$4.2 billion (2000–2010) $7.4 billion (2011–2015) $9.3 billion (2016–2020) $16.0 billion (2021–2025) $1.5 billion (2026–2037)

continued

TABLE 5-1 Continued

Type of Financing Modality	Examples	Year of Inception	Overview	Level of Funding
	Partner Contributions, Pandemic Influenza Preparedness (PIP) Framework	2011	Annual contributions from influenza vaccine, diagnostic, and pharmaceutical manufacturers that use the WHO Global Influenza Surveillance and Response System (GISRS) are pooled under a formula agreed upon by industry representatives. Partner contributions, which can fluctuate annually, are used to fund inter-pandemic preparedness efforts at the country and regional levels (70 percent) and response activities during a pandemic (30 percent).	US$227.7 billion (2012–June 2021), or approximately $28 million annually
Liability insurance	COVAX Facility no-fault compensation program for COVID-19 vaccines	2021	WHO and Chubb Limited (NYSE: CB), through ESIS Inc., a Chubb company, signed an agreement on behalf of the COVAX Facility on February 17, 2021, for the administration of a no-fault compensation program for the 92 LMICs and economies eligible for support via the Gavi COVAX Advance Market Commitment of the COVAX Facility. This is the first and only vaccine injury compensation mechanism operating on an international scale. This offers eligible individuals in eligible countries and economies a process to receive compensation for rare but serious adverse events associated with COVAX-distributed vaccines until June 30, 2022. It aims to significantly reduce the need for recourse to courts, a potentially lengthy and costly process.	US$8.3 billion (AMC for 92 LMICs)

to health security (Boyce et al., 2021), and the fund is the largest multilateral provider of grants for health system strengthening.

New and evolving financing arrangements during the COVID-19 pandemic illustrate what funding might be available, without significant changes in governance and financing instruments, for an influenza pandemic. COVID-19 funding can be loosely broken apart into investment to support preparedness or response, although those categories overlap somewhat.

COVID-19: Funding for Preparedness

One month after WHO formally declared COVID-19 a Public Health Emergency of International Concern (PHEIC), its Contingency Fund for Emergencies and the United Nations (UN) Central Emergency Response Fund allocated just $23.9 million; 3 months later, the UN Global Humanitarian Response Plan remained only 5 percent financed. The World Bank's Pandemic Emergency Financing Facility's Cash Window did not trigger until 3 months after the PHEIC was declared and was inadequate for the COVID-19 response. The full $196 million insurance payout was released in late April 2020, but it was shared among 64 countries; 59 already had management programs. Other international facilities later came into play, such as the International Monetary Fund's (IMF's) Rapid Financing Instrument and Rapid Credit Facility, which provide emergency lending to eligible countries, and, according to a paper commissioned by the IPPPR, largely fulfilled their stated objectives to contain an outbreak with pandemic potential. However, the major barrier was the lack of facilities that were ready to fill the financing gap during the earliest days and weeks of a pandemic (Radin and Eleftheriades, 2021).

COVID-19: Funding for Response

Adequate response to a pandemic requires mobilizing billions of dollars to execute well-prepared response plans at short notice. Within 6 months of the COVID-19 PHEIC declaration, more than $70 billion were committed to LMICs through multilateral agencies, with an additional $50 billion disbursed from multilateral agencies to partners. But because greater than 90 percent of these funds were in the form of debt, wealthier middle-income countries—which have greater borrowing capacities—tended to receive more funds from multilateral agencies than poorer countries (Radin and Eleftheriades, 2021). Moreover, most of this funding was directed at mitigating the broader socioeconomic consequences of the health crisis rather than at addressing the crisis itself.

In terms of vaccine development and procurement specifically, an estimated $13 billion has been invested by governments and philanthropic institutions to develop, produce, and purchase COVID-19 vaccines other than China's. The Biomedical Advanced Research and Development Authority (BARDA) grants and advance market commitments alone exceeded $10 billion (Chagar et al., 2021; Sabin-Aspen Vaccine Science and Policy Group, 2021). As of May 2021, total funding for COVID-19 vaccines and treatments had reached $119.1 billion across 277 initiatives—51.6 percent of which is country specific, and 48.4 percent multi-region.

OWS represents the largest global effort for COVID-19 vaccines. As of June 2021, OWS had invested an estimated $18 billion, much of which was channeled into late-stage clinical development and early manufacturing. Agreements were put in place to buy 455 million doses to distribute in the United States. During the same period, CEPI invested just $1.4 billion to support COVID-19 vaccines. In contrast to recipients of OWS funding, who are committed only to the United States, CEPI's funding is associated with recipients' commitments to promote global access and ensure affordable costs. Manufacturers are directly approaching countries and organizations, creating a "complicated ecosystem for COVID-19 vaccines that is comprised of a patchwork of countries that have and do not have vaccines" (Kim et al., 2021, p. e1017). In the United Kingdom and the European Union, the Oxford-AstraZeneca vaccine development was funded almost exclusively by governments or foundations. Similarly, the German government contributed $445 million to Pfizer-BioNTech's vaccine (Ramachandran et al., 2021).

However, as discussed at the beginning of this chapter, this financing has been inadequate to ensure timely global access to vaccines. According to the Rockefeller Action Plan for Financing Global Vaccination and Sustainable Growth (published in April 2021), ACT-A and COVAX will deliver 2 billion doses by 2021, but this rate (20 percent) is insufficient, and these initiatives face a shortfall of $22.1 billion. Even with a $12 billion infusion from the World Bank, The Rockefeller Foundation has argued that "the world needs to aim higher" (The Rockefeller Foundation, 2021). In spite of investments in developing COVID-19 vaccines and broadening access to them, the demand for multilateral development bank financing during the pandemic has generally been slow (Glassman, 2021). The Rockefeller Foundation has called for the use of instruments such as IMF's special drawing rights to fill financing gaps in terms of long-term pandemic response. Similarly, the Center for Global Development has proposed creating a multilateral vaccine purchase window within IMF's rapid financing instrument/concessional equivalent (rapid credit facility) (Hicklin and Brown, 2021).

New regional partnerships have recently been forged with the aim of filling the void left by COVAX's budgetary shortfalls. For instance, the

COVID-19 African Vaccine Acquisition Task Team, the Africa Medical Supplies Platform, and the Africa Centres for Disease Control and Prevention (CDC) began a COVID-19 vaccines preorder program in 2021 for all African Union (AU) member states. Afreximbank will facilitate payments by providing advance procurement commitment guarantees of up to US$2 billion to the manufacturers on behalf of the AU member states.

FINANCING PPR: ECONOMIC PRINCIPLES

Our recommendations for expanding and coordinating investment in PPR do not require arcane economic reasoning but are based on broad lessons from the COVID-19 pandemic and basic economic principles.

The key economic lessons are that pandemics can still happen in modern times despite medical and communications advances, they can explode rather than sputter out, and exploding can lead to almost *incalculable social costs*. Added to the enormous toll due to death and illness are the output losses as economies are shut down to mitigate the health losses. The U.S. Congressional Research Service (CRS, 2021) estimated that COVID-19 reduced global economic growth in 2020 to an annualized rate of -3.4 to -7.6 percent, with global trade falling by 5.3 percent. Major advanced economies may operate below their potential output level through at least 2024, with the local economic fallout leading to the worst unemployment levels since the Great Depression.[1]

Basic economics propounds the principle of *return on investment*. According to this principle, projects are not worth undertaking if they do not generate sufficient benefits in excess of expenditures. On the other hand, investments that generate large benefits at moderate expense are particularly attractive. The principle holds true for consumers deciding whether to purchase a new appliance and firms deciding whether to enter a new line of business and also for societies—individual countries or international groups—deciding whether to undertake a new program. Prior to COVID-19, HICs may have considered the small benefit of quelling an exotic epidemic disease in the developing world only worth a fraction of a small aid budget. COVID-19 now shows that the losses are more in line with those that defense and health programs are designed to avoid, justifying much higher spending levels. The principles do not imply that countries should spend the whole of their defense or health budgets on PPR—this would only be justified if pandemics were certain to happen every year. However, the possibility that pandemics may arise every one or two decades may justify spending some fraction of these budgets.

---

[1] This section is meant to be grounded in explaining the econometrics point of view, which the committee is not necessarily endorsing.

Return on investment is a rational way to increase the urgency of investment. Yet, governments, industry, and international finance institutions do not operate on purely rational terms, particularly in the realms of global public goods and preparedness—both of which are difficult to measure and quantify. Norms can be a powerful force to support international coordination and take advantage of positive externalities, as evidenced by efforts in other areas, such as the International Whaling Commission moratorium on commercial whaling in 1982. The world needs to advance its norms related to the scale of investment for PPR. Such norms may support PPR, even if they may not be relied on in the "crisis mode" of an ongoing pandemic. As described in Chapter 1, the window of political will for rethinking global investment strategies and establishing new norms concerning global public health may close quickly after the world's recovery from the COVID-19 pandemic.

Sands and others (2016b) note that infectious disease crises can cause immense economic disruption, yet mainstream macroeconomic forecasting consistently underestimates the risk. This results in underinvestment in PPR. The authors attributed this to the absence of readily available input data for such analyses and suggested an approach by which the global health community could help develop such inputs and a framework to use them in assessing economic vulnerability of individual countries and regions to infectious disease crises. They argued that incorporating these risks in influential macroeconomic analyses, such as the reports from IMF's Article IV consultations, rating agencies, and risk consultancies, would improve economic risk forecasting and reinforce government and donor incentives to mitigate infectious disease risks.

Another reason for historically low spending may be that investment in pandemic preparedness has aspects of a global public good. Research and development (R&D) grants by one country produce knowledge and new products that benefit all. Other countries have an incentive to save on grant spending by free riding on the investment of others. The epidemiology of disease spread and mutation means that disease may not be quelled anywhere unless quelled everywhere. The interconnectedness of the global economy may mean that even a country with low infection rates may continue to experience a recession if its trading partners are suffering from an outbreak. A country with adequate vaccine capacity may not be able to run it—or factories for any other products—if global supply chains are knotted up by a pandemic. The World Bank Group (2019) dubs pandemic preparedness the "ultimate" public good: it is non-excludable, is non-rival, and provides benefits to countries across the world. Economic logic says that countries only considering their individual interests will underinvest in public goods unless active measures are taken to agree on a better solution. For pandemic response, this may call for an international agreement, asking participating countries to boost spending—for example, through public policy legislation and taxation.

Even if the whole world were coordinated in a single country, pharmaceutical manufacturers and other firms in a free market could not be counted on to provide an adequate level of investment for an output, such as pandemic preparedness, due to the large *gap between social and commercial incentives*. We mentioned global social benefits from of a course of COVID-19 capacity estimated to be more than $5,000 (Kremer, 2021). However, the private value and return on investment for the companies actually installing this capacity does not match the social value. As noted by Michael Kremer, firms earned $6–$40 for a course of COVID-19 vaccine, orders of magnitude less than the social benefit. Competition and private information about benefits restrain the prices firms can charge. High prices are repugnant to consumers, and may spur regulation in ordinary times, but that is especially acute during a crisis. These forces are understandable, but reduced return on investment leads, by the aforementioned principle, to less investment and production. That repugnance during a pandemic may lead to acute undersupply. With firms rarely able to charge anything close to the social value, pharmaceutical companies should be offered substantial government incentives that are creatively structured to avoid getting the most value for spending—for example, through AMCs (Kremer, 2021).

Another relevant economic principle is the value of *early investment*. Due to compound interest, saving $100 per year for 10 years leads to a larger account than $1,000 saved in year 10. Investing before a pandemic has similar compound returns. Expanding vaccine capacity slowly during times of no disease pandemics can be much cheaper, avoiding price spikes, supply chain disruptions, and out-and-out stockouts of needed inputs. Forces for nationalizing resources present during a crisis are absent during times of no disease pandemics and may accumulate to an adequate level that can then serve the globe during crises.

Behavioral economics emphasizes the importance of *salience* to decision making. Rational computations based on deaths and other adverse events do not necessarily drive investments or shape decision making. (See the discussion of antimicrobial resistance and the O'Neill Report in Chapter 1.) Vocal supporters are a crucial catalyst in spurring investment, as evident in the relative wealth of funding for HIV and dearth of funding for efforts to combat influenza, noncommunicable diseases, and antimicrobial resistance. Momentum may also be an issue. As described in Chapter 1, the window of political will for rethinking global investment strategies may close quickly after the world's recovery from the COVID-19 pandemic.

IPPPR'S ARGUMENT ABOUT PPR FINANCING

IPPPR's *Financing Pandemic Preparedness and Response* report made a compelling case for financing PPR outside of the traditional voluntary and overseas development assistance channels (Radin and Eleftheriades, 2021). The logic is consistent with many of the economic principles laid out in the previous section. The report notes that PPR benefits are experienced globally, so it is insufficient to manage a global public good exclusively at a national level.

However, the international system lacks the financing architecture to adequately coordinate and accelerate investment in the global public goods required to contain outbreaks. HICs have largely deprioritized PPR investments and relegated these to discretionary aid, even though these countries have the most to lose economically. HICs' higher funding capacities and higher economic benefits from ending a pandemic can justify asking them to contribute more, even a *higher share* of their incomes, to finance this type of public good. It should not be financed through aid budgets. These investments should be a policy priority because they generate such large positive externalities for the entire world. Effective coordination of these investments would be a helpful "nudge" to HICs and generate large benefits, in contrast to other investments that they would make anyway.

The IPPPR report authors argue that during the COVID-19 pandemic, the main non-vaccine-specific financing gaps were in the areas of preparedness and early response, during the first 100 days from transition from outbreak to pandemic. They also argue that numerous global institutions are capable of supporting—or upscaling support for—PPR. On the vaccine front, these include CEPI and its capacity for R&D, ACT-A, including COVAX for pooled procurement, WHO's Emergency Program for technical support and operational capacity, and the Bill & Melinda Gates Foundation (BMGF), Gavi, and regional organizations such as the Africa CDC for coordinating delivery. Thus, there is no need to establish new institutions; what is needed is improved coordination and scale of financing.

SCALE OF INVESTMENT NEEDED TO IMPROVE GLOBAL PPR

Before and after the COVID-19 pandemic, studies developed estimates about the scale of investments needed to demonstrably improve PPR response worldwide. All of those studies underscore the importance of billions of dollars more in annual investments and improved coordination for the allocation and monitoring of funding; Table 5-2 provides an overview of the proposed quantities of funding. However, none of those studies looked specifically at influenza.

TABLE 5-2 Proposed Quantities of Funding Needed for Pandemic Preparedness

Proposed Plan	Funding Estimates
Rockefeller Plan (2021)	**$44 billion** through IMF Special Drawing Rights (SDRs) for COVID-19 to achieve a 70 percent vaccination rate in LMICs by the end of 2022 **$650 billion** in SDRs to catalyze an inclusive, sustainable global recovery in LMICs at no additional cost to wealthy nations
Craven et al. (2020)	**$357 billion over 10 years** estimated to build five epidemic preparedness pillars **$85–$130 billion over 2 years** for ramp-up phase to close epidemic preparedness gaps, followed by steady-state funding of $20–$50 billion annually • "Always on" systems: $56 billion • Disease surveillance: $96 billion • Prevention agenda: $88 billion • Health care capacity: $54 billion • Research and development: $62 billion
Independent Panel for Pandemic Preparedness and Response (IPPPR, 2021)	**$5–$10 billion/year** for preparedness **$50–$100 billion** in a crisis distributed by an international pandemic-financing facility
High-Level Independent Panel on Financing the Global Commons for Pandemic Preparedness and Response (HLIP, 2021)	**$15 billion/year** increase in international financing (public funding) for pandemic preparedness and response 1 percent GDP increase for LMICs for public health spending over the next 5 years
Global Health Risk Framework, National Academies of Sciences, Engineering, and Medicine (2016)	**$4.5 billion/year** committed by G7, G20, and UN to mobilize incremental financial resources Independent assessment in 2017 and every 3 years thereafter to monitor progress of implementation for upgrading public health systems, the cost of enhancing WHO's PPR capabilities, and proposed incremental investment in research and development
World Bank (2012)	**$1.9–$3.4 billion/year** for preparedness in One Health systems to bring the global zoonotic disease prevention and control system up to World Organisation for Animal Health and WHO standards, depending on disease prevalence

Preparedness-Focused Investments

In 2016, the Global Health Risk Framework made a case for investing in pandemic preparedness, which recommended that the G7, G20, and UN should commit to mobilizing incremental financial resources required—estimated to be at least US$4.5 billion per year—and monitoring the progress of implementation by an independent assessment in 2017 and every 3 years thereafter (NASEM, 2016; Sands et al., 2016a).

In May 2021, McKinsey estimated that five epidemic preparedness pillars could be built over 10 years at a cost of $357 billion (Craven et al., 2020). The report calls for a ramp-up phase to close gaps—at an estimated $85–$130 billion over 2 years—followed by steady-state funding of $20–$50 billion annually. Financing estimates for five pillars include the following:

1. **"Always on" systems,** including border health, supply chain preparation and global stockpile, emergency operations, communication and messaging, regular simulations and cross-sector exercises: $56 billion total
2. **Disease surveillance**, including pathogen surveillance and sequencing ($48 billion), U.S. national public health institutes ($3 billion), specialized surveillance programs ($4 billion), notifiable-disease and Integrated Disease Surveillance and Response-like surveillance ($19 billion), population-representative surveillance foundation ($19 billion), and data integration ($4 billion): $96 billion total
3. **Prevention agenda,** including global immunization, limited human-wildlife interactions, mapped global virome, and containing antimicrobial resistance: $88 billion total
4. **Health care capacity,** including assessing gaps in health care systems and closing pandemic-specific gaps: $54 billion total
5. **R&D,** including new antiviral, antibody, and vaccine platforms ($6 billion); scaled vaccine manufacturing capacity ($42 billion); closing known vaccine and therapeutic gaps ($14 billion): $62 billion total

The IPPPR report proposed an International PPR Financing Facility to raise additional reliable financing for pandemic preparedness and rapid surge financing for response in a pandemic (Radin and Eleftheriades, 2021). Over the long term (10–15 years), this would require $5–$10 billion per year for ongoing preparedness, providing the ability to disburse up to $50–$100 billion at short notice. This single instrument would effectively finance two windows: (1) stable long-term cash flows for capacity and (2) front-loading financing that could kick in within 2 weeks to contain an outbreak through prearranged operational response plans.

In July 2021, the G20 High-Level Independent Panel on Financing the Global Commons for Pandemic Preparedness and Response's (HLIP's) report, *A Global Deal for Our Pandemic Age*, called for $75 billion over the next 5 years in international financing for PPR, to plug major existing gaps. This would represent at least doubling current spending levels and be targeted to four gaps: infectious disease surveillance, resilience of national health systems, global capacity to supply and deliver vaccines and other medical countermeasures, and global governance. The High Level Independent Panel underscores that these costs are "negligible" compared to those of a major pandemic.

Response-Focused Investment

Response-focused investment spans both short- and long-term response. Investment in short-term response includes both preparedness and the first few months of a response phase. For instance, the IPPPR facility is designed such that international finance institutions and multilateral and regional bank capital would kick in after 3–4 months, with the ability to cover months 3–18 of a pandemic (Radin and Eleftheriades, 2021). Proposed investments in a longer-term response include the Rockefeller Plan (2021), which called for $44 billion through IMF Special Drawing Rights for COVID-19; this plan could potentially be replicated in another pandemic scenario (The Rockefeller Foundation, 2021).

STRATEGIES TO DRIVE INVESTMENT IN INFLUENZA PREPAREDNESS AND RESPONSE: ENGAGING HIGH- AND MIDDLE-INCOME COUNTRIES

PPR are public goods that are not most effectively funded by development aid. Thus, it is critical to bring HICs and middle-income countries to the table to drive investments in both preparedness—such as surveillance, vaccine R&D, and keeping facilities warm—and response. The latter includes both early and longer-term response to finance vaccine production at the scale required and then to procure and deploy the vaccines. The entire world will not be able to invest in PPR—particularly in components such as R&D and surveillance (Stutzman et al., 2020)—because LICs have opportunity costs. Ideally, countries would contribute their own funding to support health systems strengthening and surveillance—for example, Ghana is seeking international awards and funding from U.S. CDC and PIP to bolster its surveillance capacities—but this is not always feasible. Therefore, in the context of PPR, HICs should make a "big bet" that is in their own self-interest, because HICs have the most to lose, economically, during a pandemic. This point was underscored by the G20 HLIP report.

Multiple studies have concluded that lack of coordination for global access to COVID-19 vaccines significantly threatens HICs' economic recovery. For example, a study commissioned by the International Chamber of Commerce Research Foundation considered the global costs for advanced economies—after their populations are fully vaccinated—due to a continued uncoordinated approach to global vaccine distribution. It estimated that the world risks a loss of global GDP of up to US$9.2 trillion in 2021 alone; advanced economies would pay 49 percent of that regardless of their own vaccination rates (Çakmaklı et al., 2021; CARE Action + Booz Allen Hamilton, 2021).

To move these efforts forward, a key question is how to coordinate and structure middle- and high-income countries' investments in this global public good, which promotes equity, in a way that makes it the most attractive to them. The approach for universal health coverage (e.g., meetings of ministers of health and finance) is unlikely to suffice, because national investments alone are not adequate for funding and coordinating global public goods. Instead, it may be best for HICs to adopt a system of assessed contributions to a major fund. The proposed International PPR Financing Facility would raise additional reliable financing for pandemic preparedness and rapid surge financing for response (Radin and Eleftheriades, 2021). Contributions to it should be based on an ability-to-pay formula, with larger and higher-income countries paying the most. These contributions would not be considered official development assistance and in addition to that type of aid. The proposed Global Health Threats Council could allocate and monitor funding from this investment. Factors for success would be a lean secretariat, coupled with a focus on working with and through existing organizations. The intent is to fill the gap in preparedness and early response for about 3–4 months, until international financial institutions and multilateral bank capital are triggered.

KEY CONSIDERATIONS IN DETERMINING SCALE AND INCENTIVES FOR FINANCING PPR

Drawing on the IPPPR and other recent reports, the committee identified five key categories to consider when determining the scale of financing and types of incentives to use for influenza and aligned pandemic vaccine financing. These categories, which span both the preparedness and response landscape, are (1) surveillance, (2) R&D, (3) manufacturing, (4) procurement, and (5) delivery and deployment. Within each category, it is important to consider what is known about influenza funding, which considerations should be taken into account when planning for future financing, and what financing structures can generate the incentives for influenza.

Surveillance

The PIP Framework's financing for surveillance is inadequate, and WHO's Global Influenza Surveillance and Response System (GISRS) has had issues securing sufficient funding. To address this shortfall, incentives should be put in place that balance local ownership with regional or global financing.

Current Funding for Influenza and Other Respiratory Pathogens

Overall, the state of funding for surveillance of influenza and other respiratory pathogens is insufficient. WHO's funding for influenza surveillance is inadequate to cover scaling up GISRS surveillance to other respiratory pathogens, and it is supplemented by relatively small streams of financing from bilateral actors and partnerships. The committee did not systematically calculate the amounts spent on surveillance at the multilateral, regional, or national levels, as doing so would require a greater degree of transparency and longer study time frame. However, it did analyze examples of influenza-specific funding by several major players, including WHO, the World Bank, The Rockefeller Foundation, and several U.S. government agencies.

The PIP Framework has a yearly budget of approximately $28 million, of which about 90 percent goes into the Partner Contribution's Preparedness and Response funds. This pool is further broken down into (1) response funds and (2) preparedness funds for use at the country and regional levels. The latter includes funds for building surveillance capacity in WHO member states (WHO, 2019). Partner Contributions are based on a formula established when the PIP Framework was launched and have remained static since. GISRS has had difficulty securing funding for its running budget of approximately $30 million per year; it has had to seek international awards through entities such as the U.S. CDC (Dauphin, 2015). OIE/FAO Joint Network of Expertise on Animal Influenza (OFFLU), the global network of expertise on animal influenzas, is a joint collaboration among the Food and Agriculture Organization of the United Nations (FAO), the World Organisation for Animal Health (OIE), and WHO. OFFLU is poorly funded, receiving support averaging around $250,000 annually between 2005 and 2015 (Dauphin, 2015).

The World Bank's Regional Disease Surveillance Systems Enhancement (REDISSE) Programs I and II are financed by a combination of International Development Association credits and grants, International Bank for Reconstruction and Development loans, and single- and multi-donor trust funds. These programs have invested in building technical capacity in LMICs (World Bank, 2020). Between 2007 and 2012, the Rockefeller Foundation's Disease Surveillance Networks Initiative also provided grants, mostly targeted regionally. This funding led to a number of smaller regional networks, including the Mekong Basin Disease Surveillance network, East African Integrated Disease Surveillance network, and Southern Africa Centre for Infectious Disease Surveillance (The Rockefeller Foundation, 2013). REDISSE provides an example of how ministries of finance can be regionally linked for surveillance activities through regional grant funding or loan obligations. The East-Africa Public Health Laboratory Networking Project (EAPHLNP, 2021) and African Integrated Disease Surveillance network also show how national laboratories can function with regional interdependence. Each has received political buy-in and guidance from the African Union.

Additional surveillance strengthening programs include the PREDICT project, which was part of the U.S. Agency for International Development's (USAID's) Emerging Pandemic Threats program. It is led by the One Health Institute at the University of California, Davis, and has worked to improve both global surveillance for pathogens with spillover potential and workforce training. It received about $200 million over 10 years (Klein, 2020). The Preventing Emerging Pathogenic Threats program has also been allocated $9.97 million over 3.5 years by the U.S. Defense Advanced Research Projects Agency (DARPA) to focus on the Lassa and Ebola viruses (UC Davis News and Media Relations, 2019).

A major gap exists between these funding streams and the financing required to ramp up investments in surveillance for epidemic preparedness. As noted, McKinsey estimated that $25–$40 billion would be needed annually for 2 years, followed by $6–$10 billion per year for steady-state functions (Craven et al., 2020). In 2020, Dobson et al. called for an estimated $22–$31 billion per year on a global scale for preparedness against zoonotic disease outbreaks. This would support initiatives to monitor wildlife trade, programs to reduce spillovers, and programs for early detection and control, among other areas (Dobson et al., 2020). Morgan et al. (2021) estimated that supporting the implementation of integrated, sustainable, country-owned systems for national surveillance would require an investment of about $1–$4 per person each year.

Considerations for Future Financing

Ensuring future financing for surveillance warrants several key considerations. A crucial lesson learned from the COVID-19 pandemic is that collecting data daily—which is not currently done for influenza and many other diseases—can be a powerful, positive incentive for investment. Additionally, funding and governance should emphasize local ownership rather than a top-down approach. Domestic financing at the local level is critical, because implementing and maintaining systems for disease surveillance cannot rely exclusively on global funds. The tendency is to focus on the genomic and centralized aspects of surveillance at the expense of on-the-ground molecular testing. Thus, financing needs to address broader steps crucial to effective surveillance systems, such as national planning for the use of those systems.

Financing Structures to Generate Incentives

Financing structures can be leveraged to generate incentives to fund surveillance systems. For example, external financing has significant positive externalities and a powerful argument for it, but this may require core funding and defined contributions for sustained investment. Attempting to fund surveillance through episodic sources, such as the World Bank's International Development Association, is problematic. An alternative option is using funds earmarked for surveillance for governmental and nongovernmental recipients (e.g., REDISSE II, Africa CDC). The Global Fund and Gavi use co-financing arrangements as a model for incentivizing domestic investment alongside external financial support. An opportunity also exists in the investments in surveillance for COVID-19, and other diseases could be leveraged as a foundation for building broader national and/or regional capabilities, including for influenza.

R&D

Pandemic vaccines require the ability to undertake R&D for new vaccines and manufacture the vaccines at scale. Dedicated push funding is required because the pull from seasonal influenza vaccines is not sufficient to drive pandemic vaccine development.

Current Funding for Influenza

Funding for platform technologies and next-generation influenza vaccines is small relative to their potential to transform the vaccine landscape (see Chapter 4). Although the Sabin-Aspen Vaccine Science and Policy Group has called for a well-funded moonshot program for a universal vaccine, this has largely not been met with commensurate financing (Sabin-Aspen Vaccine Science and Policy Group, 2019). The most substantial investments are from HICs and high-income regions, such as the United States and the European Union. CEPI has made significant strides in forging alliances for financing and coordinating R&D for new vaccines to prevent and control infectious diseases during epidemics. However, CEPI's mandate is mainly focused on developing vaccines in the early stages, through Phase

II clinical trials, and influenza is not in its portfolio. New solutions are needed to fund high-cost, late-stage development (Sabin-Aspen Vaccine Science and Policy Group, 2019).

On the positive side, some political buy-in exists for the universal influenza vaccine. The U.S. National Institutes of Health's National Institute of Allergy and Infectious Diseases (NIAID) 2018 strategic plan highlights its commitment to support the research needed to advance the development of a vaccine that provides long-lasting protection against multiple strains for seasonal and potentially pandemic influenza (Erbelding et al., 2018). The strategy notes that "advances in influenza virology, immunology, and vaccinology make the development of a 'universal' influenza vaccine more feasible than a decade ago" (Erbelding et al., 2018, p. 347) due to efficiencies and insights in deep-gene sequencing and advances in structural biology, among other scientific innovations. In September 2019, the Trump administration issued an executive order directing the U.S. Department of Health and Human Services to modernize production by supporting the development of new manufacturing technologies for more robust and longer-lasting vaccines against a broader range of influenza viruses (Schnirring, 2019).

Although the committee did not systematically compile financial data, it identified illustrative examples of the current scale of funding for influenza vaccine R&D. The U.S. government spends \$250–\$300 million annually on influenza research, in addition to further spending on related programs, such as biodefense and biotechnology (Sabin-Aspen Vaccine Science and Policy Group, 2019). The European Innovation Council Accelerator Pilot has invested €148 million in 36 companies, including for the multi-season universal influenza vaccine OXIVAX (European Commission, 2021). As of 2019, the European Union had also funded initiatives for novel influenza vaccine development through the seventh Framework Programme for Research and Technological Development (FP7) and Horizon 2020, its research and innovation program. FP7 funded 25 influenza vaccine projects for about €87 million; an additional €18 million was granted under Horizon 2020 (Navarro-Torné et al., 2019), which also established a new influenza research partnership with India that includes matched financing (Press Trust of India, 2018).

In 2018, BMGF launched a \$12 million Universal Influenza Vaccine Development Grand Challenge with the goal of identifying

> novel, transformative concepts that will lead to the development of universal influenza vaccines offering protection from morbidity and mortality caused by all subtypes of circulating and emerging (drifted and shifted) Influenza A subtype viruses and Influenza B lineage viruses for at least three to five years.

Pilot grants ranging from $250,000 to $2 million were awarded by BMGF and the Flu Lab—an influenza-focused charitable organization—with the aim of starting clinical trials by 2021 (Sabin-Aspen Vaccine Science and Policy Group, 2019). The Wellcome Trust supported the development of CIDRAP's R&D roadmap to accelerate progress toward development of universal or broadly protective influenza vaccines (Sabin-Aspen Vaccine Science and Policy Group, 2019).

Considerations for Future Financing

Multiple considerations should be taken into account to secure future financing for influenza vaccine R&D. A 2016 WHO consultation on Global Action Plan on Influenza Vaccines (GAP I–II) identified a host of challenges related to current financing mechanisms, which underscore the need for the industry to create stronger incentives—and secure substantially more funding—to push the development of platform technologies and universal vaccines (Røttingen, 2016). Specifically, long-standing challenges for influenza vaccines include the lengthy and costly business of failure. Bringing new products to launch can take more than a decade and cost at least $1 billion—yet, at the outset, the chance of success is just 5 percent. U.S. public funding for rapid R&D response capabilities is insufficient and heavily reliant on BARDA. Furthermore, developing novel-antigen, novel-platform, broad-spectrum vaccines is hampered by many technical and regulatory challenges. Thus, a core challenge is to find ways to incentivize a smooth and sustainable shift of R&D efforts and know-how from a relatively stable market of current seasonal vaccines to a more uncertain market of pandemic and universal vaccines (Røttingen, 2016).

Funding structures for next-generation research targets are often not flexible enough to allow quick pivoting or redirection of resources. GloPID-R highlighted this barrier, which is a particular challenge for the rapid mobilization of research funds and resources, early engagements with ethics committees, and adaptive studies and trial design (Norton et al., 2020). In its 2020 background paper focused on financing pandemic preparedness R&D, the Global Preparedness Monitoring Board (GPMB)—a joint effort of the World Bank and WHO—similarly emphasized the need for major national research organizations and their governments to improve funding for collaborative R&D (World Bank Group, 2019).

Financing Structures to Generate Incentives

Financing structures that could generate incentives for R&D include push and pull funding mechanisms and structured funding. COVID-19 economic models have found that push incentives—such as direct-cost reimbursement—were hindered by funders' lack of visibility into firms' private cost information (Snyder et al., 2020). However, push funding could be used for early influenza vaccine dosing trials. For example, during the 2018 yellow fever epidemic, Brazil reduced the vaccine dose to one-fifth—in accordance with WHO's advice—which accelerated deployment. Evidence is promising that this approach might be effective for SARS-CoV-2, which could also be an analog for an influenza vaccine. For influenza, some evidence indicates that reducing the dose of an interim musculature shot or switching to intradermal could be effective strategies for vaccine dose-stretching (Kremer, 2021).

Economic modeling has demonstrated that pull incentives awarding advance purchase agreements to bidding firms were effective for late-stage vaccine development (i.e., Phase III clinical trials and manufacturing) during COVID-19 (Snyder et al., 2020). The optimal pull programs incentivized participation of nearly all the pharmaceutical firms involved in developing 10 COVID-19 viable candidates, nearly doubling the net benefits generated from the free market. AMCs can be an effective pull funding mechanism when the target is sufficiently defined. An AMC works by reducing risks—it defines the target vaccine minimum standards (efficacy, public health impact), total AMC market size, contract price, and predicted demand. Innovators and firms are assured of a subsidized price if they develop a product meeting standards and can agree to abide by affordable prices even after the AMC is depleted. Donors or country government funders are assured that funds will only be used if a highly valuable product is developed, that a competitive market is established for firms, and that their up-front investment results in sustainable supply after the AMC is depleted. Although it is not yet clear that the influenza target is well defined, working toward a universal vaccine should be a priority.

There is a strong economic case for middle-income countries, such as Russia and China, to invest in influenza vaccine R&D (Yang, 2021). The GPMB suggested several mechanisms for structured funding of vaccine development—albeit not influenza specific (World Bank Group, 2019). The first is to establish CEPI-like mechanisms for diagnostics and therapeutics to jump-start product development. This could be accomplished by new entities, an expanded CEPI structure, or an expansion of structures like GloPID-R. The second is to create research funders preposition funds—for example, through a multi-donor trust fund at the World Bank—that can be released to research organizations within days to kick-start essential research when an outbreak occurs. Additionally, the World Bank could add a senior health scientist to its own leadership to spearhead its initiatives to strengthen R&D preparedness during inter-pandemic periods. The third suggestion is that "no regret" funding should be always available to incentivize at-risk R&D before a PHEIC is declared. This amount should be reasonable to spend or lose, even if an outbreak does not expand to a major epidemic or pandemic.

Manufacturing

The next pandemic will not necessarily be caused by an influenza virus—it might even be a pathogen currently unknown to cause human disease (i.e., "Disease X"). Thus, vaccine manufacturing networks should not focus exclusively on influenza. This will require garnering broader investment in pathogen R&D alongside a universal influenza vaccine and establishing incentives for rapid scale-up of production capacity. It could be possible to create a ranked system of regionalized manufacturing centers aligned with existing agreements for clinical trials.

Current Funding for Influenza

It is critical to explore strategies for keeping mRNA and other platform technology manufacturing processes warm between pandemics for both influenza and coronavirus vaccines. The Pandemic Preparedness Partnership, launched by the UK government, prepared a report for the 2021 G7, mapping a 100 Day Mission to respond to future threats by embedding pandemic-ready manufacturing processes and capacity into business as usual (PPP, 2021). The report identifies multiple opportunities to leverage expanded vaccine production capacity between pandemics to justify maintaining surge capacity—for instance, via mass adult vaccination campaigns for various diseases, including influenza and coronaviruses. However, as discussed in Chapter 4, mRNA/platform technology mapping for influenza demonstrates that the current system for keeping facilities warm is ill prepared for these rapidly evolving new technologies. Moreover, there remains no clear cost estimate for achieving an ever-warm state for influenza vaccine platform technology, which warrants urgent research.

Considerations for Future Financing

Considerations related to future financing to keep vaccine production systems warm between pandemics are influenced by the current impetus toward distributed manufacturing, for both influenza and other pathogens with pandemic potential. However, it is important to carefully consider the distributed manufacturing business model, rather than merely distributing for the sake of doing so. If the desired outcome is to administer the greatest number of vaccines to the most people as quickly as possible, the best strategy may not necessarily require excessive differentiation between consolidated and distributed manufacturing. For example, if the United States had the entire global vaccine capacity and had immunized its population first, this might have only delayed global distribution by a few weeks. The more effective solution might involve early investment in critical technology that is generating returns, thus reducing scarcity of vaccines and associated products.

For suppliers of lifesaving materials, the general rule of thumb is at least five different manufacturers in at least five different locations. Regional and international collaborations can bolster efforts to create more diversified configurations of vaccine manufacturing, thereby promoting equity. For instance, the goals of the Africa Union Partnership for African Vaccine Manufacturing, launched in April 2021, include (1) developing a coordinated manufacturing agenda across the continent, (2) bolstering five regional partnership production sites over 10–15 years, (3) mobilizing financing, (4) strengthening regional regulation systems, (5) increasing technology transfers, and (6) developing African universities as R&D hubs (Jerving, 2021).

Most pressingly, in a distributed context, incentives need to be established to build the demand and expand the market for pandemic vaccines, because the private market alone will likely be insufficient to meet demand. Analyses of emerging infectious disease vaccines typically show that under realistic financing assumptions, expected returns are significantly negative (Vu et al., 2020).

Financing Structures to Generate Incentives

To keep vaccine manufacturing facilities warm between pandemics, several options for financing structures can generate market incentives. One strategy is to subsidize dormant capacity directly; however, maintaining facilities on standby is an expensive option. Another approach is to use manufacturing capacity for seasonal influenza to produce pandemic vaccines, although relying exclusively on this option is less viable as the system transitions away from egg-based technologies. A third option is to use the manufacturing capacity for other respiratory infections or diseases, such as adult vaccination for seasonal influenza or tuberculosis. This may be a more effective option in the shift to more versatile platform technologies.

Procurement and Access

For vaccine procurement and access, a future COVAX-like facility for influenza or other pandemic-potential pathogens should be designed with a focus on ensuring that it is resilient to deep political pressures.

Current Funding for Vaccine Procurement

Vaccine procurement methods fall into three main categories: self-procurement, donations through international organizations, and interstate procurement. Within the self-procurement approach, a government purchases vaccines from manufacturers directly on the open market. This method typically allows states to independently select the manufacturer of their choice. Although the negotiation process can result in lower prices per unit, this approach requires specialized technical knowledge in medicine and law, the financial resources necessary, a certification process for licensing vaccine safety and efficacy, and the downstream-appropriate cold-chain infrastructure to store and deliver vaccines. Some self-procuring states use advance purchase agreements (APAs), which are contracts between a manufacturer and the government that lie dormant and unenforceable until triggered by a predetermined event, when they become legally binding. The second method is to procure through international organizations (sometimes called "pooled co-procurement"), in which nongovernmental and intergovernmental organizations, such as Gavi, UNICEF, and WHO, acquire vaccines, typically through tiered pricing, and countries pay a percentage of the cost through co-financing. This approach can support providing vaccines to LICs lacking the capacity to self-procure. In some cases, the organizations procure and administer the vaccines directly if the state lacks the infrastructure. AMCs can fall under and support this mechanism; for example, the G7 and BMGF committed to buy a vaccine against LMIC-specific strains of pneumococcal disease when this vaccine was developed.

The third method involves the interstate sale of vaccines. This approach is relatively rare, but it was used during the 2009 H1N1 influenza pandemic (Turner, 2016). During that pandemic, HICs mostly used self-procurement, while LICs tended to depend on donations through international organizations. Of the more than 634 million doses obtained, almost 60 percent were via central government purchases, nearly 30 percent from other sources, and only about 12 percent deployed internationally through donations to WHO's Vaccine Deployment Initiative, which was created specifically to manage the distribution of vaccines then (see Chapter 2). That 12 percent of donated vaccines accounted for about 94 and 91 percent of the African and Southeast Asian regions' vaccines, respectively. Self-procurement was heavily associated with HICs—nearly 99 percent of vaccines in the European region were acquired through self-procurement, compared to just 6 percent in Africa. In a case study of vaccine procurement during the 2009 pandemic, Eccleston-Turner maintains that these methods were ineffective for developing states and predicts that during the next influenza pandemic, global demand for vaccines will exceed the worldwide supply, which is dominated by developed states with existing APAs (Turner, 2016).

Similar trends have emerged during the COVID-19 pandemic. HICs have cornered the vaccine market through APAs with prices that are heavily dependent on individual procurement contracts. Only a relatively small percentage of vaccines are donated or sold to international organizations for allocation to LMICs through entities such as COVAX. Even before vaccines were authorized and approved, many countries entered into bilateral bulk purchasing agreements with individual manufacturers to secure doses at lower negotiated prices. For instance, through two separate agreements, Moderna secured a $3.2 billion contract to provide the United States with 200 million doses at roughly $16 per dose; the European Union secured doses from Moderna at $18 per dose. Pfizer also received two separate contracts for a total of 200 million doses at $19.50 per dose, while the European Union paid just under $15.15 (Ramachandran et al., 2021).

However, prices of vaccines may not reflect a fair return on public investments in vaccine R&D, and these types of "competitive pricing" could quickly make vaccines unaffordable for LMICs. At a 2020 hearing of a U.S. House Oversight and Investigations Subcommittee, leading manufacturers were asked whether they would supply COVID-19 vaccines at cost or no profit. Only two—AstraZeneca and Johnson & Johnson—stated that they would be willing to do so for a limited number of doses or during "the emergency pandemic period." Both Pfizer and Moderna said that they would not. Further uncertainty is fueled by the lack of clarity around how to define the "pandemic period" during which companies have promised to supply their products at lower prices or to share technology with other manufacturers. Although AstraZeneca pledged not to profit from its vaccine during the pandemic period, the company also specified that it could declare the pandemic over by July 2021. Pharmaceutical executives have stated they anticipate returning to "commercial pricing" as early as late 2021, and Pfizer has already raised the prices of the European Union's future orders by more than 60 percent (Ramachandran et al., 2021).

In early March 2021, COVAX declared its intention to make 1.8 billion doses available to countries with AMCs by the end of 2021, which would cover an estimated 28 percent of those countries' populations (Hall et al., 2021). In the interim, some LMICs and regions have used self-procurement. However, this has exacerbated problems related to manufacturers charging customers different prices for the same product. For example, according to a senior health official in South Africa, the country purchased 1.5 million doses of the Oxford/Astra-Zeneca vaccine for health workers at $5.25 per dose, more than double the price ($2.15 per dose) for the European Union. This price disparity emerged only due to inadvertent disclosures, as the European Union had kept its prices confidential in exchange for vaccine discounts. The South African Deputy Director-General of Health said his government had been told that $5.25 was the set price for a country classified by the World Bank as upper middle income (Dyer, 2021).

Figure 5-3 provides an overview of COVID-19 vaccine supply agreements by country and group, illustrating the extent to which APAs have dominated the market, often leaving behind LMICs. For instance, COVAX collectively procured approximately the same percentage of vaccines as the United States has individually, as of June 2021. UNICEF has tracked reported COVID-19 vaccine prices per dose, which demonstrates how the procurement system has led to wide variances in cost (for the same vaccines) for different customers (see Figure 5-4).

Considerations for Future Financing

The global distribution of seasonal influenza vaccines remains highly inequitable across regions. The PIP Framework's procurement system for LMICs covers just a small percentage of the total vaccine capacity, so a new COVAX-like procurement and access facility will likely be required to ensure that countries in the WHO Eastern Mediterranean, South East Asia, and Africa Regional Offices have access. Between 2004 and 2017, the share

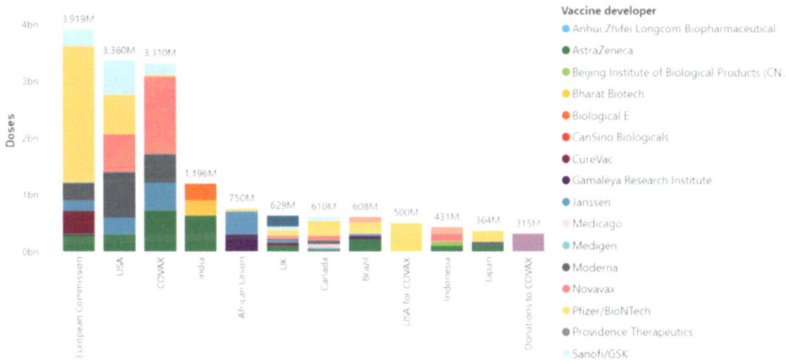

FIGURE 5-3 COVID-19 vaccine supply agreements (doses) by recipient country/group.
SOURCE: https://www.unicef.org/supply/covid-19-vaccine-market-dashboard (accessed December 19, 2021).

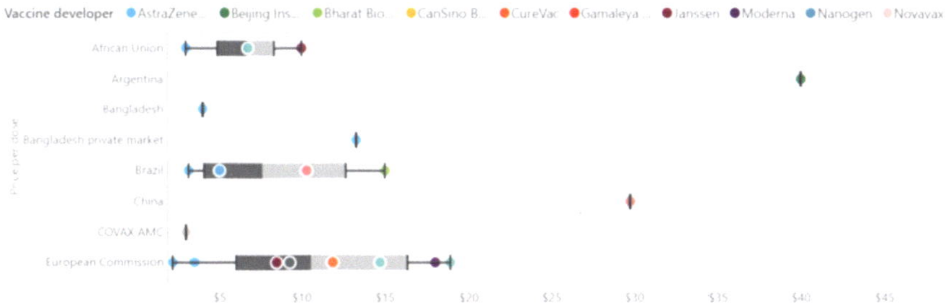

FIGURE 5-4 Reported COVID-19 vaccine price per dose.
SOURCE: https://www.unicef.org/supply/covid-19-vaccine-market-dashboard (accessed December 19, 2021).

of seasonal doses increased in the Americas (41–55 percent) and declined in both Europe (34–22 percent) and the Western Pacific (24–17 percent). In Africa, the Eastern Mediterranean, and Southeast Asia, the combined share of doses increased from 5 to 6 percent. The latter is unacceptably low, given that these regions represent almost half of the world's population (Sparrow et al., 2021). Furthermore, in determining the optimally equitable distribution, it is important to consider economic losses in addition to death rates.

The COVID-19 pandemic has demonstrated that theoretical models for effective and equitable delivery may not stand up to political pressure. Efforts by COVAX and other entities to improve global access were undermined by vaccine nationalism; amid the chaos of competing priorities, HICs tended to embrace bilateral deals that would allow for scale-up. Successful incentives to promote equitable distribution must be catalyzed by political commitments and supported by mechanisms and models of cooperation that can withstand political pressure.

Game theory analyses have identified two ways that mechanisms such as COVAX can shape incentives to promote scale-up and broaden global access to vaccines. The first is to leverage self-enforcing good behavior norms, global prestige, and social sanctioning. This approach is based on articulating principles of how countries ought to structure bilateral deals and transparency. The second strategy is to create extra benefits that only those making equitable or "good" deals can enjoy (McAdams et al., 2020). There have been calls to create separate versions of COVAX-like mechanisms for different diseases and expand existing facilities to vaccines against pandemic pathogens. However, it is difficult to predict the type of pandemic that is likely to strike next and important to design a platform specific to the immediate situation.

Financing Structures to Generate Incentives

Appropriate financing structures can generate procurement incentives and promote equitable access worldwide. For example, vaccine supplies for LICs should be included as components of grants and contracts with vaccine developers, as CEPI did with some manufacturers for COVID-19. This should be done before Phase III trials, when efficacy will be established and global demand will be high. Furthermore, providing up-front, at-risk manufacturing to global procurers, such as Gavi and the Global Fund, can enable large-volume pre-purchasing, as done by both the United States and the United Kingdom during COVID-19.

After its inception in 2016, CEPI developed an equitable access policy with input from key stakeholders and formed an Equitable Access Committee as a subcommittee of the CEPI Board. Early in the COVID-19 pandemic, CEPI included clauses in partnering agreements with vaccine manufacturers that included a manufacturing component to secure doses for "a global procurement and allocation entity" that had not yet been developed. CEPI has sought to enable low pricing by requiring developers to enter into procurement deals with Gavi for COVAX. In such cases, the price is determined by negotiations between the developer and Gavi on behalf of the facility. In addition, CEPI has the right to redirect the supply to another public-sector procurer. All the agreements require compliance with CEPI's equitable access policy and/or contain similar commitments in principle, including pricing at levels that are affordable to the people who need the vaccines (CEPI, 2021). This provides a model for how future equitable access clauses may be built into AMCs for influenza vaccines.

Delivery and Deployment

Although delivery and deployment of vaccines ("vaccination") faces serious challenges—particularly in LICs—the financing for this is often overlooked.

Current Funding for Influenza

Delivery is often an underconsidered and underresourced cost, yet it can be more substantial than the cost of vaccine production. CARE estimates that countries or donors should invest $5 in delivery for every $1 invested in COVID-19 vaccine doses (Janoch et al., 2021). Although the delivery cost of influenza vaccines globally during a future pandemic has not been clearly quantified, estimates of the delivery component's cost for COVID-19 may be instructive.

McKinsey has reported that during COVID-19, far less has been invested in planning for and implementing country vaccine rollout than for procurement. According to COVAX reports, in-country rollout costs about $1.50 per dose for delivery to the first 20 percent of the population, which does not include the health care workforce required. COVAX would only be able to provide a small percentage of this cost. An estimated $1 per dose—about $1.3 billion—would need to come from other domestic, bilateral, and/or multilateral sources. The World Bank's $12 billion lending programs could theoretically help provide vaccine delivery support, but countries may not choose this borrowing mechanism (Hall et al., 2021).

A report from UNICEF, WHO, Gavi, BMGF, Harvard, ThinkWell, and the World Bank experts estimated that delivering COVID-19 vaccines to approximately 20 percent of the population in the 92 AMC countries would cost $2.018 billion—including country, regional, and global costs—about $1.66 per dose or $3.70 per person vaccinated with two doses (COVAX Working Group on Delivery Costs, 2021). Of this total cost, 57 percent is in-country outreach and fixed site delivery costs and 28 percent is country up-front fees (e.g., cold-chain installation, training). The report notes that delivery costs will vary substantially based on a range of factors, including specific target groups, population outreach strategies, geography, and local prices.

Another analysis estimated that about $74 billion would be required to reach COVID-19 vaccine herd immunity in LMICs—67 percent of this ($50 billion) for procurement and 33 percent ($24 billion) for delivery. This delivery cost is prohibitive for many countries; an estimated 20 percent of LMICs would have a total vaccine cost that is at least 10 times higher than their baseline annual immunization spending (Mustafa Diab et al., 2021).

Considerations for Future Financing

In considering financing strategies for vaccine delivery and deployment, a key lesson from the COVID-19 pandemic and other recent outbreaks is that most countries are far from adequately prepared to deploy critical medical supplies to their populations at the breadth and speed required. Health systems in LMICs typically lack capacity to deal with infectious diseases—particularly providing adult vaccines. In HICs, infectious disease control also tends to be a weak point in otherwise strong health systems. Successful responses to outbreaks tend to occur more often in countries with relatively strong existing health systems and recent infectious disease experience, such as Vietnam.

Furthermore, it is not efficient to create exclusively influenza-specific systems (e.g., cold chains, workforce). Thus, efforts to strengthen delivery and deployment capacity should build on and expand existing influenza frameworks such that they can be leveraged for a range of respiratory pathogens. Vaccine hesitancy continues to hinder influenza vaccine uptake, but local manufacturing capacity and stronger regulatory structures could increase local trust.

COVID-19 revealed the absence of an entity responsible for ensuring that liability policies and vaccine injury compensation programs were in place before the vaccine. However, COVAX did create a new program to compensate eligible individuals in 92 LMICs without requiring legal processes. The program, funded by a small levy on each dose, is the first and only vaccine injury compensation mechanism established on a global scale. Only 25 countries, including the United States and wealthier regions within Asia and Europe, have mechanisms to compensate individuals who receive serious vaccine-related injuries for routinely recommended vaccines (Sabin-Aspen Vaccine Science and Policy Group, 2021).

Financing Structures to Generate Incentives

Linking preparedness for influenza and other pathogens of pandemic potential to endemic diseases could help to increase national funding, including for deployment. Ideally, deployment strategies would not be specific to influenza. For example, they could cover other adult vaccinations, including COVID-19 boosters, in line with the WHO Immunization Agenda 2030, which emphasizes the importance of vaccination across the lifespan. External deployment financing should be channeled to support national vaccination and pandemic plans—particularly with the support of large nongovernmental organizations, such as the Bangladesh Rural Advancement Committee in Bangladesh, and through existing international organizations with experience in vaccine deployment–related planning, implementation, supply chains, and monitoring, such as UNICEF and Gavi.

KEY FINDINGS AND CONCLUSIONS

Surveillance Financing

- Surveillance system gaps are related both to financing and to barriers for more closely aligning or integrating these systems. They are far from being an LMIC problem; many HICs have moved away from financing surveillance systems efficiently, and many financed systems underperform in terms of accuracy, scope, and transparency. This is at least in part due to lack of political buy-in and country leadership.
- Domestic and external funding, accompanied by synchronous laws and legal instruments, may enable national surveillance systems to be more regionally operational and interdependent (e.g., sharing technical expertise, capital goods, operating expenditures, and information).
- The amounts and allocation of funding for surveillance should be sufficient to develop integrated surveillance systems that include all forms of influenza (human and animal) at a minimum and, ideally, include other respiratory pathogens with pandemic potential.
- Surveillance is primarily a global risk mitigation—not a development—issue. The economic theory argument is very compelling for surveillance of influenza and other pathogens with pandemic potential.
- While surveillance is a "best buy" in terms of cost-effectiveness, strengthening surveillance systems requires more than incentives. Each country's surveillance system generates strong positive externalities

that benefit all countries. This makes surveillance an area where there is a strong logic for sustained domestic and external financing. It should therefore not compete with other development priorities.

R&D, Manufacturing, and Procurement Financing

- For influenza and other pathogens with pandemic potential, industry is often insufficiently certain of the government interests and regulatory pathway to bring a profitable product to the market.
- A concerted effort is needed to demonstrate the direction that pharmaceutical companies should be moving in within the influenza space, toward transformation next-generation technologies and universal influenza vaccine targets.
- A moonshot for universal influenza vaccines should be initiated to support a portfolio of next-generation/platform vaccines, which would offer higher efficacy and the potential for a more sustainable business model for scale-up. Such an effort should benefit from and include a similar quest for more broadly protective ("variant-proof") vaccines against coronaviruses with pandemic potential.
- The scale of investment in universal influenza vaccines to date (millions) is nowhere near the scale required (billions) to incentivize the risky undertaking of such R&D.
- Both push and pull incentives will be critical to demonstrate a proof of concept for the market of influenza vaccines. A massive push will be required to elicit pre-competitive scientific and biological analyses for influenza vaccine targets. AMCs (pulls) have most commonly been used by HIC donors to incentivize vaccine production and capacity for proven vaccine approaches, rather than to drive new science. AMCs can be usefully deployed as an incentive to solve hard biology problems such as those implicit in a universal influenza vaccine.
- Universal influenza and platform technology push and pull instruments should include equitable access provisions, in line with CEPI's model during the COVID-19 pandemic.

Markets and Deployment

- The scalability of influenza vaccines is limited by the number of companies and production processes and by limited markets where the burden of this illness is uncertain.
- A vaccine market supported by an immunization program able to deliver vaccines, coupled with a population demand for these vaccines, are essential elements to ensure a sustainable vaccine manufacturing base.

- Stronger national plans for deploying seasonal influenza vaccines (using next-generation/platform technologies) and recognizing that vaccines will increasingly be available across the lifespan (in line with the WHO Immunization Agenda 2030) are essential for vaccine markets and have a strong public health rationale.
- Deployment activities require proper technical guidance and designated financial resources, but care should be taken to not frame deployment as a positive externality. Vaccine deployment requires designated financing from high- and middle-income countries according to a Global Public Good framework and also national accountability.
- UNICEF and Gavi have decades-long experience in deployment planning, implementation, supply chains, monitoring, and policies. Both are well positioned to take the lead on global coordination for vaccine deployment, particularly in LMICs.

REFERENCES

Boyce, M. R., A. Attal-Juncqua, J. Lin, S. McKay, and R. Katz. 2021. Global Fund contributions to health security in 10 countries, 2014–20: Mapping synergies between vertical disease programmes and capacities for preventing, detecting, and responding to public health emergencies. *Lancet Global Health* 9:e181–e188. https://www.thelancet.com/journals/langlo/article/PIIS2214-109X(20)30420-4/fulltext (accessed August 22, 2021).

Burwell, S., F. Townsend, T. Bollyky, and S. Patrick. 2020. *Improving pandemic preparedness: Lessons from COVID-19.* Council on Foreign Relations Independent Task Force Report Number 78. https://www.cfr.org/report/pandemic-preparedness-lessons-COVID-19/pdf/TFR_Pandemic_Preparedness.pdf (accessed October 25, 2021).

Çakmaklı, C., S. Demiralp, Ş. Kalemli-Özcan, S. Yeşiltaş, and M. A. Yıldırım. 2021. *The economic case for global vaccinations: An epidemiological model with international production networks.* Cambridge, MA: National Bureau of Economic Research. https://www.nber.org/system/files/working_papers/w28395/w28395.pdf (accessed October 25, 2021).

CARE Action + Booz Allen Hamilton. 2021. *The case for U.S. investment in global COVID-19 vaccinations.* https://www.care.org/wp-content/uploads/2021/04/The-Case-for-U.S.-Investment-in-Global-COVID-19-Vaccinations-Policy-Paper.pdf (accessed December 19, 2021).

CEPI (Coalition for Epidemic Preparedness Innovations). 2021. *Enabling equitable access to COVID-19 vaccines: Summary of equitable access provisions in CEPI's COVID-19 vaccine development agreements.* https://www.readkong.com/page/enabling-equitable-access-to-covid-19-vaccines-summary-of-4837506 (accessed October 25, 2021).

Chagar, A., M. Thomas, L. Zuo, and M. Watson. 2021. *The R&D response to COVID-19: What can we learn for the vaccine ecosystem?* Sabin-Aspen Vaccine Science and Policy Group. https://www.kearney.com/documents/20152/134482507/THE+R%26D+RESPONSE+TO+COVID-19.pdf/4ff5d86b-fa90-c542-33ba-1fa2deb9f46e?t=1621954683000 (accessed October 25, 2021).

Cohen, J., and K. Kupferschmidt. 2021. Fairer shares. *Science* 372(6545):903.

COVAX (COVID-19 Vaccines Global Access) Working Group on Delivery Costs. 2021. *Costs of delivering COVID-19 vaccine in 92 AMC countries.* https://www.who.int/publications/m/item/costs-of-delivering-covid-19-vaccine-in-92-amc-countries (accessed December 19, 2021).

Craven, M., A. Sabow, L. Van der Veken, and M. Wilson. 2020. *Not the last pandemic: Investing now to reimagine public health systems.* McKinsey Report. https://www.mckinsey.com/industries/public-and-social-sector/our-insights/not-the-last-pandemic-investing-now-to-reimagine-public-health-systems (accessed October 24, 2021).

CRS (U.S. Congressional Research Service). 2021. *Global economic effects of COVID-19.* Report R46270. Updated July 9, 2021. https://crsreports.congress.gov/product/pdf/R/R46270 (accessed July 16, 2021).

Dauphin, G. 2015. Coordination tripartite OMS/FAO/OIE pour le contrôle et la prévention des virus influenza zoonotiques. Illustration avec OFFLU, réseau mondial d'expertise vétérinaire. *Bulletin de l'Académie Vétérinaire de France* 224.

Dobson, A. P., S. L. Pimm, L. Hannah, L. Kaufman, J. A. Ahumada, A. W. Ando, A. Bernstein, J. Busch, P. Daszak, and J. Engelmann. 2020. Ecology and economics for pandemic prevention. *Science* 369(6502):379–381.

Dyer, O. 2021. COVID-19: Countries are learning what others paid for vaccines. *BMJ* 372:n281.

Erbelding, E. J., D. J. Post, E. J. Stemmy, P. C. Roberts, A. D. Augustine, S. Ferguson, C. I. Paules, B. S. Graham, and A. S. Fauci. 2018. A universal influenza vaccine: The strategic plan for the National Institute of Allergy and Infectious Diseases. *The Journal of Infectious Diseases* 218(3):347–354.

European Commission. 2021. *EU research and innovation supporting vaccine development for COVID-19.* https://op.europa.eu/en/publication-detail/-/publication/69212491-6f3d-11eb-aeb5-01aa75ed71a1 (accessed December 19, 2021).

Glassman, A. 2021. *Money in the bank: What's behind slow demand for MDB financing for vaccines?* https://www.cgdev.org/blog/money-bank-whats-behind-slow-demand-mdb-financing-vaccines (accessed June 16, 2021).

Hall, S., L. Kaplow, Y. S. Sun, and T. Z. Holt. 2021. *"None are safe until all are safe": COVID-19 vaccine rollout in low- and middle-income countries.* McKinsey and Co. https://www.mckinsey.com/industries/healthcare-systems-and-services/our-insights/none-are-safe-until-all-are-safe-covid-19-vaccine-rollout-in-low-and-middle-income-countries (accessed October 24, 2021).

Hicklin, J., and H. Brown. 2021. *Vaccine financing: How a redesigned IMF instrument can provide a shot in the arm for the global pandemic response.* Washington, DC: Center for Global Development.

HLIP (High-Level Independent Panel). 2021. *A global deal for our pandemic age: Report of the G20 High-Level Independent Panel on Financing the Global Commons for Pandemic Preparedness and Response.* https://pandemic-financing.org/report/foreword (accessed October 24, 2021).

IPPPR (Independent Panel for Pandemic Preparedness and Response). 2021. *COVID-19: Make it the last pandemic.* https://theindependentpanel.org/wp-content/uploads/2021/05/COVID-19-Make-it-the-Last-Pandemic_final.pdf (accessed December 19, 2021).

Janoch, E., M. Rodriguez, and B. Turner. 2021. *Our best shot: Women frontline health workers around the world are keeping you safe from COVID-19.* https://www.care.org/news-and-stories/health/our-best-shot-women-frontline-health-workers-around-the-world-are-keeping-you-safe-from-covid-19 (accessed October 24, 2021).

Jerving, S. 2021. *AU launches partnership for African vaccine manufacturing.* https://www.devex.com/news/au-launches-partnership-for-african-vaccine-manufacturing-99654 (accessed April 14, 2021).

Kim, J. H., P. Hotez, C. Batista, O. Ergonul, J. P. Figueroa, S. Gilbert, M. Gursel, M. Hassanain, G. Kang, B. Lall, H. Larson, D. Naniche, T. Sheahan, S. Shoham, A. Wilder-Smith, N. Strub-Wourgaft, P. Yadav, and M. E. Bottazzi. 2021. Operation Warp Speed: Implications for global vaccine security. *The Lancet Global Health* 9(7):E1017–E1021. https://www.thelancet.com/journals/langlo/article/PIIS2214-109X(21)00140-6/fulltext (accessed December 19, 2021).

Klein, A. 2020. *This won't be the last pandemic. Where will the next one come from? New Scientist.* https://www.newscientist.com/article/2246259-this-wont-be-the-last-pandemic-where-will-the-next-one-come-from (accessed October 24, 2021).

Kremer, M. 2021. *Presentation at National Academy of Medicine international workshop on COVID-19 lessons to inform pandemic influenza response.* https://nam.edu/event/international-workshop-on-covid-19-lessons-to-inform-pandemic-influenza-response-day1 (accessed October 24, 2021).

McAdams, D., K. K. McDade, O. Ogbuoji, M. Johnson, S. Dixit, and G. Yamey. 2020. Incentivising wealthy nations to participate in the COVID-19 vaccine global access facility (CooV): A game theory perspective. *BMJ Global Health* 5(11):e003627.

Morgan, O. W., X. Aguilera, A. Ammon, J. Amuasi, I. S. Fall, T. Frieden, D. Heymann, C. Ihekweazu, E.-k. Jeong, G. M. Leung, B. Mahon, J. Nkengasong, F. N. Qamar, A. Schuchat, L. H. Wieler, and S. F. Dowell. 2021. Disease surveillance for the COVID-19 era: Time for bold changes. *The Lancet* 397(10292):2317–2319.

Mustafa Diab, M., A. Zimmerman, S. Dixit, W. Mao, I. Bharali, A. Kristoffersen, G. Yamey, and O. Ogbuoji. 2021. The cost of procuring and delivering COVID-19 vaccines in low- and middle-income countries: A model of projected resource needs. http://dx.doi.org/10.2139/ssrn.3824690 (accessed October 25, 2021).

NASEM (National Academies of Sciences, Engineering, and Medicine). 2016. *Global health risk framework: Pandemic financing: Workshop summary.* Washington, DC: The National Academies Press.

Navarro-Torné, A., F. Hanrahan, B. Kerstiëns, P. Aguar, and L. Matthiessen. 2019. Public health–driven research and innovation for next-generation influenza vaccines, European Union. *Emerging Infectious Diseases* 25(2):e180359. https://wwwnc.cdc.gov/eid/article/25/2/18-0359_article#suggestedcitation (accessed October 25, 2021).

Norton, A., L. Sigfrid, A. Aderoba, N. Nasir, P. G. Bannister, S. Collinson, J. Lee, G. Boily-Larouche, J. P. Golding, E. Depoortere, G. Carson, B. Kerstiëns, and Y. Yazdanpanah. 2020. Preparing for a pandemic: Highlighting themes for research funding and practice—perspectives from the Global Research Collaboration for Infectious Disease Preparedness (GloPID-R). *BMC Medicine* 18(1):273.

PPP (Pandemic Preparedness Partnership). 2021. *100 days mission to respond to future pandemic threats.* https://assets.publishing.service.gov.uk/government/uploads/system/uploads/attachment_data/file/992762/100_Days_Mission_to_respond_to_future_pandemic_threats__3_.pdf (accessed December 19, 2021).

Press Trust of India. 2018. *India, EU to develop new influenza research programme named Horizon 2020; pay €15 million each to fund project.* https://www.firstpost.com/india/india-eu-to-develop-new-influenza-research-programme-named-horizon-2020-pay-e15-million-each-to-fund-project-5063951.html (accessed October 25, 2021).

Radin, E., and C. Eleftheriades. 2021. *Financing pandemic preparedness and response.* Independent Panel for Pandemic Preparedness and Response, Background Paper 14. https://theindependentpanel.org/wp-content/uploads/2021/05/Background-Paper-14-Financing-Pandemic-Preparedness-and-Response.pdf (accessed October 25, 2021).

Ramachandran, R., M. Dhodapkar, J. S. Ross, and J. L. Schwartz. 2021. Future of COVID-19 vaccine pricing: Lessons from influenza. *BMJ* 373:n1467.

The Rockefeller Foundation. 2021. *One for all: An action plan for financing global vaccination and sustainable growth.* New York: The Rockefeller Foundation.

Røttingen, J.-A. 2016. *Alternative models for influenza vaccine R&D financing.* Presentation by CEPI at the third WHO consultation on Global Action Plan on influenza vaccines (GAP III). https://www.who.int/influenza_vaccines_plan/GAPIII_Session4_Rottingen.pdf (accessed October 25, 2021).

Sabin-Aspen Vaccine Science and Policy Group. 2019. *Accelerating the development of a universal influenza vaccine.* https://www.influenzer.org/app/uploads/2020/01/sabin-aspen-report-digital.pdf (accessed October 25, 2021).

Sabin-Aspen Vaccine Science and Policy Group. 2021. *Powering vaccine R&D: Opportunities for transformation.* https://www.aspeninstitute.org/wp-content/uploads/2021/05/Sabin-Aspen-Report-2021.pdf (accessed October 25, 2021).

Sands, P., C. Mundaca-Shah, and V. J. Dzau. 2016a. The neglected dimension of global security—a framework for countering infectious-disease crises. *New England Journal of Medicine* 374(13):1281–1287.

Sands, P., A. El Turabi, P. A. Saynisch, and V. J. Dzau. 2016b. Assessment of economic vulnerability to infectious disease crises. *The Lancet* 388:2443–2488.

Schnirring, L. 2019. *Trump signs executive order to improve flu vaccines.* https://www.cidrap.umn.edu/news-perspective/2019/09/trump-signs-executive-order-improve-flu-vaccines (accessed October 25, 2021).

Snyder, C. M., K. Hoyt, D. Gouglas, T. Johnston, and J. Robinson. 2020. Designing pull funding for a COVID-19 vaccine. *Health Affairs* 39(9):1633–1642.

Sparrow, E., J. G. Wood, C. Chadwick, A. T. Newall, S. Torvaldsen, A. Moen, and G. Torelli. 2021. Global production capacity of seasonal and pandemic influenza vaccines in 2019. *Vaccine* 39(3):512–520.

Stutzman, H., A. Micah, and J. Dieleman. 2020. *Funding pandemic preparedness: A global public good.* https://www.thinkglobalhealth.org/article/funding-pandemic-preparedness-global-public-good (accessed October 25, 2021).

Turner, M. 2016. Vaccine procurement during an influenza pandemic and the role of advance purchase agreements: Lessons from 2009-H1N1. *Global Public Health* 11(3):322–335.

UC (University of California) Davis News and Media Relations. 2019. *$9m to preempt zoonotic spillover threats, protect military and local communities.* https://www.ucdavis.edu/news/9m-preempt-zoonotic-spillover-threats-protect-military-and-local-communities (accessed October 25, 2021).

Vu, J. T., B. K. Kaplan, S. Chaudhuri, M. K. Mansoura, and A. W. Lo. 2020. *Financing vaccines for global health security.* National Bureau of Economic Research, working paper 27212. https://www.nber.org/papers/w27212 (accessed October 25, 2021).

WHO (World Health Organization). 2019. *Partnership Contribution (PC) Preparedness High-Level Implementation Plan II 2018–2023, revised version.* Geneva, Switzerland: World Health Organization.

WHO. 2021a. *WHO chief warns against "catastrophic moral failure" in COVID-19 vaccine access. UN News January 18, 2021.* https://news.un.org/en/story/2021/01/1082362 (accessed July 22, 2021).

WHO. 2021b. *Director-General's opening remarks at the World Health Assembly—24 May 2021.* Geneva, Switzerland: World Health Organization https://www.who.int/director-general/speeches/detail/director-general-s-opening-remarks-at-the-world-health-assembly---24-may-2021 (accessed July 22, 2021).

WHO. 2021c. *Joint COVAX statement on supply forecast for 2021 and early 2022.* Geneva, Switzerland: World Health Organization. https://www.who.int/news/item/08-09-2021-joint-covax-statement-on-supply-forecast-for-2021-and-early-2022 (accessed October 25, 2021).

World Bank. 2020. *Epidemic preparedness and response.* https://www.worldbank.org/en/results/2020/10/12/epidemic-preparedness-and-response (accessed October 25, 2021).

World Bank Group. 2019. *Pandemic preparedness financing: Status update.* https://www.worldbank.org/en/search?q=Pandemic+preparedness+financing%3A+Status+update (accessed October 25, 2021).

Yang, S. 2021. *Rising-power competition: The COVID-19 vaccine diplomacy of China and India.* Emerging Voices on the New Normal in Asia. National Bureau of Asian Research. https://www.nbr.org/publication/rising-power-competition-the-covid-19-vaccine-diplomacy-of-china-and-india (accessed October 25, 2021).

6

Recommendations and the Path Forward

SITUATING INFLUENZA IN THE BROADER PANDEMIC PREPAREDNESS AND RESPONSE CONTEXT

Efforts to strengthen global coordination, partnerships, and financing for pandemic and seasonal influenza vaccines are an integral and essential part of the world's overall efforts to reinforce these for the level of pandemic preparedness and response (PPR) needed to address any pandemic threat. A significant window of opportunity exists now to strengthen the world's overall PPR architecture. For example, the Independent Panel for Pandemic Preparedness and Response (IPPPR), G7/UK International Pandemic Preparedness Partnership (PPP), G20 High-Level Independent Panel on Financing the Global Commons for Pandemic Preparedness and Response (HLIP), and proposals for a pandemic treaty or instrument, have all been active in 2021. Preparing for influenza as one of, but not the sole, major pandemic threat recognizes that, epidemiologically, seasonal influenza imposes a major, annual societal burden across countries during non-pandemic years and that this family of viruses also causes influenza pandemics, which could disrupt society as much or more than any other known microbiological threat.

The core requirements for strengthening national and global influenza PPR systems and capabilities are foundational for the PPR agenda, including surveillance, pathogen sharing, vaccine technologies, manufacturing capacity, intellectual property (IP), regulatory issues, and vaccine delivery (which encompasses vaccine acceptance and demand for a broader range of microbiological threats). An influenza pandemic is an essential PPR scenario for which national authorities must plan. Given historical patterns, the present and known existence of specific influenza viruses of concern, ongoing conditions that favor the emergence of another influenza pandemic, and the severe global experience with COVID-19, it is incumbent on decision makers to materially strengthen PPR broadly and influenza PPR specifically. It is important to undertake this in a way that reduces the health and public health consequences of pandemics caused by influenza and other pathogens and acknowledges their economic and societal impact.

While integrating such efforts into the broader PPR agenda makes sense, we must also recognize two points. First, the starting point with influenza is different from that/those for other pathogens; well-established, although underfunded, networks and legal arrangements exist to meet the twin challenges of seasonal and pandemic influenza, and especially the frequent need to update the antigenic composition of vaccine. These provide systems that, in concept, can be extended to include other pathogens (as has already happened with Global Influenza Surveillance and Response System [GISRS] with regard to SARS-COV-2), although the uniqueness of different pathogens also means that such extensions cannot be achieved blindly. It is essential to ensure that integration into the broader agenda does not undermine what is already working well in existing influenza-focused networks. Second, like all pathogens, influenza has distinctive characteristics, of which the most striking are the following:

- The influenza viruses creating predictable, annual "seasonal" epidemics of disease and also some spilling over from their normal animal hosts to become infectious in, and transmissible among, humans at unpredictable times;
- The limited global use of antiviral therapeutics and diagnostic tests, underscoring the importance of vaccines;
- The well-established and relatively well-understood and monitored nature of the zoonotic links, compared to many other emerging infectious diseases; and
- The long historical pattern of pandemics, including the 1918–1919 pandemic, and the capacity of influenza viruses to cause another highly severe pandemic.

Acknowledging and acting on the core principle of fair and equitable access to vaccines is a required foundation for broad and sustained support for the global coordination mechanisms and agreements necessary for a PPR agenda for respiratory pathogens, including vaccines for pandemic influenza. There are two complementary ways to approach equitable allocation of vaccines: creating specific frameworks that include equity considerations directly and scaling up and distributing manufacturing to reduce scarcity.

International or regional frameworks can strengthen global coordination and time lines, while national plans are necessary to ensure nationally and locally appropriate approaches for vaccine deployment and vaccination. However, the COVID-19 pandemic has underscored that even access and benefit-sharing (ABS) agreements alone might not be adequate to counter vaccine nationalism. The Pandemic Influenza Preparedness (PIP) Framework, in particular, is untested and, in its current form, would not provide timely and equitable quantities of vaccines for low- and middle-income countries (LMICs). The COVID-19 experience suggests that the scalability, size, and sustainability of the vaccine supply is an important complementary requirement to strengthen equitable access to vaccines under urgent conditions and ensure that vaccine manufacturing capacity and immunization programs are able to reach those at highest risk. In this context, acceptance of the principles of equity and fostering of innovation are twin pillars.

Governance innovations for influenza vaccines are therefore necessary. These vaccines have severe constraints on production capacity and time lines, including those related to the present dominance of egg-based methods. Investment in multiple platforms will benefit the timely availability of adequate amounts of influenza vaccine under pandemic conditions. While at least 22 (see Table 4-1) COVID-19 vaccines have been produced, scaling up influenza capacity requires platform technologies. Improving influenza vaccines' breadth of protection (efficacy and ability to protect high-risk groups) and duration of protection must also be a priority, especially given the impact they have already demonstrated. Above all, a dedicated and well-resourced effort to develop a universal influenza vaccine that can provide durable protection against any influenza virus that is capable of causing serious human infections could take the threat of influenza—both seasonal and pandemic—off the table.

The importance of scaling up surge manufacturing capacity for influenza vaccines cannot be overstated. Any significant global rationing of limited vaccine capacity during a future pandemic will inevitably lead to a repeat of vaccine nationalism. More geographically distributed vaccine manufacturing might help somewhat in terms of ensuring that particular countries or geographic regions have access to vaccines but will not automatically lead to equitable allocation. Places that gain manufacturing capacity may well behave in ways similar to existing manufacturing hubs, resulting in *distributed vaccine nationalism*, which is better than the status quo but probably still leaves the poorest countries and communities at acute disadvantage. The *realpolitik* of pandemic politics suggests that actors in the G7 and G20, such as the United States, that possess vaccine manufacturing facilities and leading-edge scientific capabilities, will remain unwilling to give up their places in the vaccine "queue." A more realistic path is to persuade such actors to make the queue move faster by investing in greater surge capacity. This core conclusion informs a number of the report's recommendations.

Achieving an equitable global allocation ultimately requires balancing global frameworks and regulations (top-down), enhanced funding for deployment and national planning (bottom-up), and supply and demand considerations (preventing scarcity). With COVID-19, this balance was not reached by high-income countries (HICs) and the number of "deals" made along the way, leading to vaccine nationalism, contracting delays, and a lack of transparency about the vaccine supply. For an influenza pandemic, creating norms through a strengthened PIP Framework or similar instrument and/or binding commitments, combined with structural solutions to reduce the period of extreme vaccine scarcity (such as procuring stockpiles and setting pre-existing procurement contracts), may allow establishing a "grand bargain." Crucially, the future business case for influenza must recognize that the seasonal influenza vaccine market alone will not be sufficient to drive pandemic production.

When approaching global coordination, partnerships, and financing for influenza and other respiratory pathogens with pandemic potential, it is vital to consider the underlying grand bargain that must be reached among stakeholders. It is based on a concept of support with obligations, or an understanding that each involved party—including but not limited to industry, sovereign states, and multilateral and bilateral agencies—should give information, products, funding, or infrastructure of value (e.g., viral sequences, obligations to build surveillance capacity, investments into new technologies). They therefore must expect to receive certain benefits (e.g., reasonable access to vaccines, funding for government investments, IP protections). In other words, a balance must be struck between multilaterals and industry contributing money or innovations and the sharing of benefits accruing from these innovations.

This grand bargain forms the centerpiece of how to respond to a global public good—and how to encourage the high- and middle-income country investments that will be required for the PPR agenda. Each recommendation in this report should be viewed according to this global public good framework, with some recommendations focusing more on ensuring that benefits are shared with member states on the medical countermeasures side (e.g., pathogen-sharing systems), others focusing more on assurances for contributors that positive externalities are delivered by member states (e.g., strings attached to global surveillance funding), and others recognizing the importance of voluntary industry partnerships (e.g., the risk of disincentivizing innovation). Given this context, the committee's core recommendations address the following:

- Significantly reinforcing global influenza surveillance as part of a broader upgrade of disease surveillance;

- Incentivizing pathogen and genetic sequence sharing (for influenza and other pathogens);
- Building a coordination structure for sustained industry partnerships to optimize companies' platform technologies for efficient vaccine production and efficacy;
- Creating a combination of push/pull incentives (e.g., advance market commitments [AMCs]) and resources to make the development of next-generation and, ideally, universal influenza vaccines a priority;
- Incentivizing the development of sustainable, geographically distributed hubs to scale up vaccine production and relevant supply chains, through a global partnership program coordinated by CEPI or another organization with a global reach;
- Ensuring that financing solutions for global surveillance encompasses all pathogens with regional or global pandemic potential, includes zoonotic components, and incentivizes pathogen and genetic sequence sharing; and
- Building demand and national pandemic and adult vaccination planning capacity by ensuring that adequate funding is available to procure, deploy, and deliver next-generation influenza vaccines to any population group identified to be at increased risk.

The precise financing vehicles for each of these elements should be solved as part of the broader PPR financing solution rather than influenza specific. Some recommendations are targeted at the G7 and G20, with the understanding that the "Global Health Threats entity" ultimately put forward by these initiatives should take a leadership role in their implementation. This should not be taken as de-emphasizing the importance of other parties, such as the "Group of 77" (G77), industry, and civil society organizations, in global negotiations and discussions, and the committee includes examples of such parties that should be involved in implementing each recommendation. In proposing the G7 and G20 Global Health Threats entity's leadership, the committee is not offering a precise view on the relative merits of the various proposals for a Global Health Threats Board or Council by the G20, G7, United States, or United Kingdom, as this involves considerations beyond its Statement of Task.

CONCLUSIONS AND RECOMMENDATIONS

1: Governance and Coordination to Support Aligned Vaccine Production and Scale-Up for Respiratory Pathogens with Pandemic Potential

Among infectious diseases, the technical and policy systems related to influenza, including for surveillance (GISRS), the vaccine strain selection process, and related ABS governance frameworks (PIP Framework) are global and relatively well coordinated through the World Health Organization (WHO). In many respects, influenza vaccine development represents a uniquely close functional relationship or ecosystem among scientists, governments, and the private sector. For example, the annual process to identify relevant strains to include in seasonal vaccines involves formal and informal discussions between public health practitioners, academics, and regulators regarding the preparation and sharing of reagents.

However, beyond the process of strain selection, the development and manufacturing processes for influenza vaccines are relatively uncoordinated and in the hands of the private sector, with wide variability across national policies and programs. This reflects differences among nations in their vaccination priorities and WHO's long-standing challenges in engagement with industry. The private sector and industry are not limited to research and development (R&D) pharmaceutical companies. In the United States and most emerging economies, including China and India, the private clinical sector is dominant, public and private health insurance companies are major policy-influencing actors (e.g., U.S. Medicare was an original major driver for influenza vaccine use), and many large universities involved in R&D are private-sector entities. Most of these fall outside the purview of WHO and even the ministries of health of other nations.

Summary of findings: Scaling up production of influenza vaccines is limited by the number of companies and production processes, limited markets where the burden of illness is uncertain, and limited coordination between the human and animal sectors. Programs supporting platform technology R&D and industry partnerships to scale up vaccine production and address supply chain chokeholds are often performed in a semi-isolated context. This is true for influenza *and* other respiratory pathogens with pandemic potential. The COVID-19 pandemic has also demonstrated that—like influenza—these other pathogens may become "endemic" such that coordination will be critical for producing, procuring, and distributing vaccines. This reinforces the need to move away from historical siloed systems toward a single architecture for the global coordination of PPR, in the spirit of the GISRS+ and Global Early Warning System for Major Animal Diseases (GLEWS+) proposals.

> **Conclusion 1A.** *Global coordination for vaccines and vaccination will not be successful without including both public (world governments) and private actors—including civil society and the pharmaceutical and biotechnology industries. WHO is well placed to provide normative guidance, technical support for integrated surveillance, and regulatory support for vaccine licensure for the coordination of global, regional,*

and national programs for PPR that recognize the importance of operating across multiple pandemic threats.

Conclusion 1B. *WHO is less well positioned to support activities that require deep engagement with the private sector and industry, including vaccine manufacturing, supply chains, and deployment across multiple pathogens with pandemic potential.*

Recommendation 1: The World Health Organization (WHO) should develop an integrated agenda to strengthen preparedness and response for all respiratory pathogens of pandemic potential, which includes surveillance, information sharing, and the development, manufacturing, and deployment of vaccines and other essential components of the vaccine manufacturing supply chain. This agenda should comprise a key component of the overarching agenda for pandemic preparedness and response, encompass pandemic influenza, and build on existing mechanisms for coordination in the influenza arena. To accomplish this, member states should task WHO to:

a. Assume leadership for this agenda and, with collaboration from relevant multilateral partners (e.g., the Food and Agriculture Organization of the United States and the World Organisation for Animal Health), propose a framework for strengthened surveillance systems and information sharing at country, regional, and global levels to ensure rapid detection of new threats and enable swift dissemination of information essential to accelerated vaccine development.

b. Work jointly with existing international and stakeholder organizations with expertise in vaccine research and development, manufacturing coordination and supply chain management, and deployment (e.g., the Coalition for Epidemic Preparedness Innovations, the United Nations Children's Fund, and Gavi, the Vaccine Alliance) to develop, in consultation with vaccine manufacturers, a framework for improved global coordination of vaccine development, production, and deployment for respiratory pathogens with pandemic potential that includes defined roles, responsibilities, and accountability mechanisms.

2: Sustainable Financing for Integrated, Modern, Timely Respiratory Virus Surveillance for Pathogens with Pandemic Potential

The ongoing and dynamic emergence and spread of coronavirus variants has reinforced that surveillance systems are critical to assess risk and serve multiple purposes for a country's priority-setting for health.

Robust and timely surveillance systems are at the heart of public health and essential for evidence-based country vaccination systems—and, more broadly, for nearly every aspect of a country's pandemic response. They provide the data and insights needed to set priorities and monitor the impact of interventions. They enable governments to know which pathogens are circulating; establish baselines of disease levels, so trends and deviations can be monitored; provide background information useful for determining the safety and efficacy of therapeutics and vaccines and predictive value of diagnostic tests; and support making disease control decisions related to outbreaks. For diseases with epidemic and pandemic potential, they provide the signals needed to act as disease early warning systems; they are the global "smoke detectors" that can keep emerging sparks from becoming a global fire. Additionally, pathogen-focused surveillance provides essential information for formulating effective vaccines and assessing the effectiveness of available treatments (e.g., antiviral drug resistance).

The concept of "surveillance" is often considered from the lens of viral data ("pathogen" surveillance), but in the twenty-first century, it also encompasses other components of early warning systems, including data on social media and human movement. Several new initiatives have been launched, based on this recognition that genomic surveillance and early warning data gathering capabilities across multiple pathogens must be built to allow the world to contain pandemic threats within 100 days of an outbreak. These include the UK Global Pandemic Radar and The Rockefeller Foundation's Pandemic Prevention Institute (The Rockefeller Foundation, 2021). Without national surveillance infrastructure and robust regional surveillance systems for both pathogens and epidemiological trends, countries are left in the dark about upcoming threats, which has massive ramifications for national, regional, and global health security. Determining how to expand funding for these surveillance activities for viruses with pandemic potential, including influenza, is therefore critical.

Summary of findings: Surveillance system gaps are related to both financing and barriers for more closely aligning or integrating these systems. They are far from being an LMIC problem; many HICs have moved away from financing surveillance systems efficiently, and many financed systems underperform in terms of accuracy, scope, and transparency. This is at least in part due to lack of political buy-in and country leadership.

Robust surveillance systems require working across traditional sector silos, particularly to identify zoonotic threats and spillover events. One of the key challenges for developing broader surveillance systems is how to cover multiple pathogens, including zoonotic surveillance for influenza, which has not been funded in a sustained way. Surveillance represents a prime example of how ministries and organizations, particularly those in the animal and health sectors, can develop misaligned objectives that contribute to silos based on competition for influence, power, and funding. It is critical for ministries of health to be joined by other relevant ministries, such as ministries of agriculture and of the interior, in surveillance programs. Ministries of the interior are often the main actors (next to prime ministers or presidents) in terms of decision-making "power" during emergencies, including pandemics. Coordination, information sharing, and collaboration among intragovernmental agencies will improve the alignment of objectives across governments.

WHO and other international organizations cannot direct national ministries to take certain steps. They can, however, offer technical and managerial guidance and support and suggest policy solutions and mechanisms to facilitate multilateral agreements at the country level and provide close follow-up. For example, the PIP Framework resulted from prolonged international negotiations within WHO, which produced an agreement that provided financial backing to member states to improve national surveillance systems that participate in the WHO GISRS network. The same agreement provided access to potential pandemic influenza viruses and the sharing of vaccines, antiviral medicines, and other benefits in a pandemic. However, the PIP Framework does not generate enough money to strengthen GISRS in all places.

Global and regional influenza surveillance should not only be enhanced to include both traditional and nontraditional data that can help to identify an emerging threat earlier but also have an overall financing solution that encompasses human and animal influenza and incorporates pathogen and genetic sequence sharing as routine practices. This will require substantially greater multilateral investments in country and global surveillance. Perhaps the most crucial premise for this is recognizing that surveillance is primarily a global risk assessment and mitigation—not a development—issue. The economic theory argument is very compelling for surveillance of influenza and other pathogens with pandemic potential. Yet, while surveillance is a "best buy" in terms of cost-effectiveness, strengthening these systems requires more than incentives. Each country's surveillance system has strong positive externalities. This makes surveillance an area with a strong logic for sustained domestic and external financing, as with France's support to the Pasteur Institutes in Africa. This funding is best conceptualized as being part of how the world as a whole addresses extreme risks. It should not be forced to compete with other development priorities.

Domestic and external funding, accompanied by synchronous, consistent, and ideally coordinated laws and legal instruments, may enable national surveillance systems to be regionally operational and interdependent (e.g., through sharing technical expertise, capital goods, operating expenditures and approaches, and information). The World Bank's Regional Disease Surveillance Systems Enhancement (REDISSE) model provides an example of how ministries of finance can be regionally linked for surveillance activities through regional grants or loan obligations (West African Health Organization, n.d.).[1] The East-Africa Public Health Laboratory Networking Project also shows how national laboratories can function with regional interdependence. Both have received political buy-in and guidance from the African Union (AU). The IPPPR and other groups are working on recommendations for institutional mechanisms for surveillance, including a global viral surveillance network. This study's findings and deliberations underscore that integrated viral surveillance should be structured to support country ownership and cover critical *influenza* data needs, including genomic sequence data and integrated zoonotic surveillance.

Enhancing surveillance systems to protect against a range of pandemic threats will require a dedicated, sustained pool of financing that can be applied nationally and regionally and does not divert funding from other development priorities. Surveillance must be viewed as an essential element to maintain public health and second-order consequences of economic and societal well-being if it is to attract sustained, stable, long-term financing. Its benefits must be framed more broadly, such as access to medical countermeasures downstream.

> **Conclusion 2.** *The amounts and allocation of funding for surveillance should be sufficient to develop integrated surveillance systems that include all forms of influenza (human and animal) at a minimum and, ideally, encompass other respiratory pathogens with pandemic potential. Others are giving financial estimates (see Chapter 5)—which we draw on—for how much should go into strengthening surveillance, and our recommendations focus on how to make certain that influenza is given sufficient weight. This funding could be used to initiate or strengthen country and regional surveillance networks, in line with the REDISSE model.*

> **Recommendation 2: With urgency (over the next 3–5 years), the G7 and G20 should ensure that increased investments are made in surveillance systems for pathogens with pandemic potential, which support and encompass every country and region, by doing the following:**
>
> **a. Creating incentives, structures, and pathways for key stakeholders to develop and implement integrated surveillance, which should include firmer support for zoonotic surveillance in the framework of One Health programs, such as through the World Health Organization (WHO), the World Organisation**

[1] See https://www.wahooas.org/web-ooas/en/projets/redisse-regional-disease-surveillance-systems-enhancement-project-west-africa (accessed December 30, 2021).

for Animal Health (OIE), and the Food and Agriculture Organization of the United Nations (FAO) stakeholders.

b. **Strengthening and financing regional surveillance structures and networks through partnerships between regional development banks and organizations. For example, in the South Asia and Southeast Asia regions this could be accomplished in conjunction with the Association of Southeast Asian Nations, Asian Development Bank, and Asian Infrastructure Investment Bank, and in the Middle East and North Africa with the Organization of Islamic Cooperation, Gulf Cooperation Council, and Islamic Development Bank.**
c. **Ensuring that the financing mechanism selected by the G7/G20 for pandemic preparedness and response more broadly includes sustainable funding for surveillance and that this pooled funding is sufficient to enable surveillance for respiratory pathogens, especially encompassing those with pandemic potential, at the national and regional levels.**
d. **This global funding mechanism's governance should include relevant international agencies, such as the International Fund for Agricultural Development, OIE, FAO, and the World Food Program, in addition to multilateral and regional development banks and WHO.**

3: Limits and Potential of the PIP Framework and Nagoya Protocol for Pathogen Sharing

The timely sharing of influenza viruses is essential for developing life-saving seasonal vaccines, identifying potential pandemic viral strains, and providing early warning for outbreaks. The PIP Framework supports critical surveillance needed for influenza and establishes a multilateral system that places equal importance on ABS and sharing viruses of pandemic potential but avoids a bilateral transactional approach to such sharing. It reflects the importance of transparency, equity, and the accountability shared by countries, industry, and WHO.

The current controversy at the World Trade Organization around the IP waiver for COVID-19 technologies is a consequence of the lack of a careful and planned approach to related ABS. The balance between virus, genetic sequence, and benefit sharing must consider public investment, global needs, and private rights and incentives, but it cannot be ignored. ABS is an essential aspect of equity and is needed to garner global support, while IP is a paramount necessity for industry's wholehearted support and ongoing investments in innovation. Momentum is building for a new pandemic instrument, providing an opportunity to incorporate diplomatic gains from earlier negotiations and agreements into new multilateral solutions. Such an instrument would eliminate the challenge of negotiating in the midst of a pandemic threat, ensuring predictability and a general mutually agreed framework and saving the critical time needed to put a full response in place. More specifically, the principles agreed upon in the PIP Framework, which are essentially consistent with those of the Convention on Biological Diversity (CBD), could be incorporated into the foundations of any future multilateral instrument for pandemics. Certain pros and cons to devising such an instrument go beyond the committee's mandate and are highlighted briefly in this chapter's final section.

Summary of findings: The PIP Framework is built on the need for transparency, equity, efficiency, and accountability of countries, industry, and WHO. Beyond access to vaccines and medicines at reduced prices, other essential benefits can include updated epidemiological information, capacity building, training, and publications. It stands in contrast to the bilateral approach espoused by the Nagoya Protocol and approaches sharing benefits according to the shared need of all countries for early warning, preparation against pandemic threats, and access to vaccines, diagnostic tests, and medicines needed to protect their populations.

However, the PIP Framework has limitations: it does not specifically cover genetic sequence data and only covers *influenza* viruses with *pandemic potential* and not seasonal influenza viruses or other viruses that might cause a pandemic. Its ability to ensure the availability of vaccines and antiviral medications under pandemic conditions and distribute them equitably remains untested and raises the question of whether the vaccine nationalism prominent early in the COVID-19 response would be repeated for an influenza pandemic. While it remains theoretically possible for the framework to be expanded to include seasonal influenza, other viruses, and genetic sequence data, WHO member states and other key stakeholders, including leading pharmaceutical companies, have not achieved consensus on the feasibility of doing so. Expanding the scope of the PIP Framework to non-influenza viruses, in particular, would raise the substantial challenge of extending its commitments of sharing, close cooperation, and division of labor in the absence of an established framework, such as GISRS.

The underlying core principles of the PIP Framework remain highly relevant and should be incorporated into a pandemic treaty or other future international instrument: (1) giving equal weight to sharing of viruses and benefits; (2) ensuring shared responsibility and accountability among countries, WHO, and the private sector (although both industry and civil society operate at the international law level through member states); (3) recognizing the fundamental importance of equity and responding to country needs, particularly for LMICs; and (4) putting WHO at the center of negotiation and making sure that benefits flow multilaterally through it and not bilaterally.

Another layer of the PIP Framework has less to do with core principles and more to do with the specific ways in which it is implemented. This layer is customizable and can be negotiated for multilateral agreements covering ABS for pathogens with pandemic potential. Three of these implementation considerations are particularly salient. First, part of the money spent on the PIP Framework is contributed by industry annually. A future multilateral agreement would need to carefully consider that platform and recombinant technologies are bringing new firms into the market, perhaps leading to no well-defined group of firms that produce influenza vaccines (with a similar trend for vaccines for other pathogens with pandemic potential). Heavily taxing industry through required shares in an ABS framework may also negatively incentivize firms to provide inputs into the vaccine system. At the same time, the financial contribution by industry to the PIP Framework reflects the benefits industry derives from participation in and maintaining an equitable and reasonable system of financial and other contributions.

Second, beyond supporting surveillance, PIP Framework funds are used to help countries and regions to develop capacities and capabilities, such as regulatory reform, that allow them to respond faster during a pandemic. The COVID-19 response has demonstrated the importance of these investments for broader PPR, and a future agreement would need to carefully consider which benefits to finance at the country level. Third, the details of benefit-sharing mechanisms, such as the legally binding standard material transfer agreements 2 (SMTA-2s), could easily change and be approached differently in a future agreement. A pandemic treaty negotiation is likely to be prolonged and take several years, and additional time would be needed for it to enter into force. Negotiations for the WHO Framework Convention on Tobacco Control (FCTC), for instance, took 4 years, had its first protocol adopted 7 years after its mother convention came into force, and took another 6 years to enter into force itself. A pandemic treaty or instrument is best viewed as a mid- to long-term systemic solution, leaving open the need for more immediately applicable mechanisms.

Delays in sharing samples, sequences, and information have serious implications for delaying a pandemic response. Every player—including National Influenza Centres (NICs), countries, vaccine manufacturers, and WHO—can exhibit both immediate self-serving and collaborative behaviors. It is therefore critical to encourage and enable rapid sharing and characterization of samples. In a pandemic, lack of timely sharing of viruses and associated information could have very serious implications for delaying the response (WHO, 2021a). Sharing genetic sequence data also has a major gap, due to an uncertainty about whether it falls under the PIP Framework and Nagoya Protocol. The rapid ramp-up of genomic surveillance for SARS-CoV-2 virus variants underscores the need to ensure rapid access to genetic information.

Conclusion 3A. *This is the time for the foundational principles of the PIP Framework to be incorporated into future multilateral agreements covering access and benefits for all pathogens with pandemic potential. Benefit sharing should be seen and acted upon as a routine responsibility of the global vaccine system and not in a narrow and transactional way or as a selective and ad hoc activity. Industry may be best incentivized to produce necessary vaccines through platform technologies and ensure that they are distributed equitably when mechanisms for ABS are visible and built into procurement contracts (i.e., with fair access principles up front).*

Conclusion 3B. *A new agreement should address and resolve issues raised by the Nagoya Protocol for sharing influenza viruses and other pathogens with pandemic potential, including genetic sequence data.*

Recommendation 3: The World Health Assembly (WHA) should explicitly clarify that the Pandemic Influenza Preparedness (PIP) Framework covers genetic sequence data. The WHA should also use established PIP Framework principles as a foundation for future World Health Organization (WHO) member state agreements, or advocate for their use in agreements negotiated by other international organizations, so that the access and benefit and information-sharing principles cover a broader range of pathogens and their genetic sequence data. To accomplish this, the WHA should, with support of the United Nations, do the following:

a. Establish accountability and compliance monitoring for member states and other parties in the PIP Framework and future agreements on access and benefit sharing (ABS) through regular reviews and meetings of member states, and by building or strengthening norms and holding leaders accountable for following through on commitments.

b. Incorporate the principles of equity, shared accountability, and multilateralism in any future pandemic treaty or instrument and ensure that the surveillance systems that can rapidly detect, assess, report, and share these viruses are publicly recognized to be a global public good.

c. Develop a mechanism for countries to share viruses openly and rapidly, including their genetic sequences and other essential supporting laboratory information and epidemiological data for both risk assessment and risk management (developing vaccines,

therapeutics, and diagnostics), while setting up incentives for industry and member states to share benefits and products (vaccines, therapeutics, and diagnostics), and to facilitate transferring technology. This requires a recognition of the concerns of industry over intellectual property. This mechanism should include regular public reporting as part of a transparency and monitoring system to hold countries and governments accountable for their level of pandemic preparedness and response.

d. Request that the WHO secretariat approach the Convention on Biological Diversity (CBD) secretariat to initiate a process for a new international agreement or instrument to be established as a "special international instrument" under Article 4.4 of the Nagoya Protocol (allowing the agreement to bypass some Nagoya Protocol requirements while remaining consistent with its objectives). The new international agreement or instrument could either be negotiated as an additional protocol to the CBD alongside the Nagoya Protocol, be a component of a possible future pandemic treaty, or be negotiated within WHO as a new ad hoc international agreement. The special international instrument should address the sharing of genetic sequence data and other necessary information, such as important epidemiological and laboratory data, in addition to the pathogen samples. The Meeting of the Parties to the Nagoya Protocol, in collaboration with WHO, should recommend that Parties to the Protocol facilitate and streamline national implementation procedures to facilitate the timely international sharing of pathogens in line with the urgency of responding to an outbreak. The Meeting should also acknowledge that genetic sequences of both human and animal pathogens are essential for modern science to adequately assess and respond to outbreak emergencies and to develop optimal vaccines, diagnostic tests, and other critical materials. Consideration should also be given to reinforcing that any ABS portion of the agreement not deter innovation or act as a disincentive for industry participation.

4: Public–Private Partnerships to Accelerate Vaccine Development: Structuring Global Partnerships to Support R&D for Influenza Platform Technologies

Vaccine development and production for pandemic influenza and emerging infectious diseases has traditionally suffered market failures, in large part because of the combined unknowns of whether (and when) a pandemic will hit and whether pandemic response products will be effective. This has created significant hurdles for vaccines, such as those for Zika and Middle East respiratory syndrome (MERS), to cross the finish line as commercial products. Seasonal influenza vaccines, and potential vaccines for endemic diseases, such as malaria and tuberculosis, provide a more certain product in terms of market predictability and certainty.

Public–private partnerships with industry before and during the COVID-19 pandemic have allowed highly efficacious platform technology–based vaccines to be developed. Platform technologies could revolutionize the effectiveness, speed, and ability to scale up production of influenza vaccines, due to intrinsic constraints with the current egg-dominated vaccine ecosystem. The strong market for COVID-19 vaccines (potentially including boosters if the disease becomes endemic) may not, however, represent a workable model for creating sustainable markets for all emerging infectious diseases and the associated vaccine R&D. Because of the high mutation rate and other characteristics of the influenza virus, developing platform technologies for pandemic and seasonal influenza viruses will require significant investment and a continued willingness of industry to form productive, synergistic partnerships.

Summary of findings: Successfully responding to the "necessity" of platform innovation for influenza vaccines requires a combination of early R&D incentives, including support of Phase I–III clinical trials for platform- and recombinant-based technologies. Vaccine manufacturers will share efficiencies of their production ("yield") but often only with partners. Encouraging and incentivizing *voluntary* industry partnerships will assist with developing platform technologies—and initiating their technology transfer—and should also be designed to support the partnerships needed for a universal influenza vaccine moonshot (see Recommendation 5).

Vaccine development and production time lines have been accelerated for other diseases through well-financed partnerships, such as Operation Warp Speed (OWS) for COVID-19, the HERA Incubator (COVID-19), CEPI's early manufacturing investments, and Gavi's AMC for pneumococcus and COVID-19 vaccines. Each of these schemes helped to spur healthy competition in developing novel vaccines, at least partly because their incentives package of R&D funding, up-front guarantees for advance purchase agreements, and technical support was applied mostly at once. Other examples of productive government–industry partnerships include DARPA's Autonomous Diagnostics to Enable Prevention and Therapeutics program, launched in 2013, which has primarily supported vaccine and antibody programs against the chikungunya virus, and the Biomedical Advanced Research and Development Authority (BARDA)-supported funding of Zika vaccine program toxicology studies, Phase 1 clinical trials, and associated manufacturing activities (awarded in 2016). Both programs supported mRNA technology development at Moderna.[2] Government involvement helps to avoid competitive issues, and government financing incentivizes industry to focus on a platform's optimization, which will likely be unique for each technology.

Such government–industry partnerships could be extended to include relevant academic organizations, scientific R&D institutes or programs, and foundations that support them (e.g., the Mo Ibrahim Foundation). Clinical trials can also be institutionalized on a stronger base through partnerships, building on existing programs (e.g., the European and Developing Countries Clinical Trials Partnership). The difficulty is in how to scale up such partnerships and apply them globally, especially to support a geographically distributed manufacturing hub model.

The Sabin-Aspen Vaccine Science and Policy Group (2019) proposed creating a new entity to support platform innovation for influenza vaccines, but at the time (2018), there was little appetite for creating a new global organization. Several existing organizations may be able to lead large-scale R&D and clinical trials for influenza platform technologies, including large-scale global action in LMICs, if they are given expanded mandates that are matched with appropriate funding and can identify stable markets for their products, including CEPI, BARDA, and the HERA Incubator. CEPI has an existing platform with scientific expertise and networks that span the first three steps in the process: preclinical development, clinical development, and scale-up. As Yamey et al. (2020) argued, adding funding for the advanced development of vaccines could provide transaction cost efficiency compared to launching a new mechanism, and large investments could allow CEPI to extend its expertise to Phase III trials and potentially technology transfer. The CEPI 2.0 agenda demonstrates CEPI's strategic interest in helping to extend platform technologies more broadly for respiratory viral families that present recurrent and critical threats, or "prototype pathogens." With its current level of funding, its interest in influenza would primarily be in developing influenza vaccine platforms as a way to situate the collective responsibility among major R&D funders (e.g., G7 and G20) and as a springboard for industry to move toward testing platforms against a range of pandemic-potential pathogens.

Fostering scale-up and promoting equity in access to products developed through these partnerships will require close collaboration with geographically distributed manufacturing hubs (see Recommendation 6). As a public–private partnership with a multilateral approach, CEPI iW well positioned to address cost-effectiveness thresholds for influenza R&D on a global scale. BARDA and HERA have similar capacities for advanced vaccine development, at the early, middle, and late stages. OWS, for instance,

[2] See https://www.modernatx.com/ecosystem/strategic-collaborators/mrna-strategic-collaborators-government-organizations (accessed December 19, 2021).

has been called a "souped-up BARDA" and is an example of what might work for influenza vaccine platform development, both for R&D and for manufacturing scalability to have surge capacity during a pandemic. OWS attributes include its strong central management, sufficient funding for its objectives, and high level of oversight. These enabled it to be involved in all operational aspects of manufacturing for Moderna's COVID-19 vaccine, including accessing and ordering raw materials, obtaining special equipment and machinery, hiring and training talent, and validating work to support scale-up (see Chapter 4). Giving BARDA a broader remit may allow it to overcome a limitation of OWS: it did not account for global need by building out the way that the United States works with industry. Additionally, it will be important to improve coordination for influenza vaccine research at CEPI and/or HERA and BARDA with institutional R&D capabilities beyond the United States, particularly in Germany (e.g., the Max Planck Institute), Japan, and South Korea, and to engage regional entities for R&D mobilization.

Encouraging governments and regional bodies to conceptualize R&D using an industrial policy framework may further promote resource allocation (staff and funding) to vaccine-related industry partnerships in the long term. Many successful East Asian economies, such as Japan, South Korea, China, Vietnam, Singapore, and Taiwan, have strong industrial policies, which could be expanded to include pandemic preparedness and R&D priority areas and may open-up the larger sources of funding required to push forward platform innovation and generate markets for emerging infectious disease vaccines.

> **Conclusion 4A.** *The goal in the next 3–5 years should be to progressively pursue development and assessment of new platform technologies to improve the effectiveness of vaccines, expand the options for production of influenza vaccines, and optimize their production to enhance the speed and volume of manufacturing in parallel to pursuing the "ultimate prize," a universal influenza vaccine. It could take the threat of influenza—seasonal and pandemic—off the table.*

> **Conclusion 4B.** *Manufacturing thought leaders from industry and academia need to develop new ways of working together to more rapidly advance new technologies and to optimize production (e.g., increasing yield efficiency) before a crisis to meet the public health goal of producing more vaccines sooner while ensuring that the process does not sacrifice safety. Because of the competitive nature of the vaccine business, this sharing should take place under the auspices of government partnerships, with appropriate intellectual property protections,*

while also recognizing the public health function of the products being developed.

Conclusion 4C. *The COVID-19 pandemic has underscored that pandemic viruses may become endemic, or linger on as "seasonal" viruses, in addition to influenza. Vaccine capacity should anticipate vaccination needs beyond a pandemic.*

Recommendation 4: The Global Health Threats Board or similar governance structure created by the G7/G20 PPR agenda, should negotiate to extend the mandates of the Coalition for Epidemic Preparedness Innovations (CEPI), the Biomedical Advanced Research and Development Authority, the HERA Incubator, and equivalents elsewhere as appropriate, to support government–industry partnerships for research and development (R&D) for influenza and other respiratory viruses with pandemic potential. These voluntary partnerships should focus on optimizing each industry partner's platform, using the following structure:

a. The G7 and G20 member nations (e.g., through the Global Health Threats Board) should name a global coordination body to specifically coordinate global and regional government–industry partnerships for influenza vaccines. CEPI is the existing multilateral global coordination vehicle for R&D, has access principles built in, and is a possible organization to assume this role.
b. Countries that fund vaccine R&D should ensure that R&D for pandemic influenza is part of their funding portfolio and strive to identify investment synergies to maximize returns on investments. Regional organizations should support the mobilization of government–industry partnerships, such as the Africa Centres for Disease Control and Prevention, the Association of Southeast Asian Nations, the Gulf Cooperation Council, and Europe 2020's Innovation Union (funded by HORIZON 2020) and its successor.
c. Government–industry partnerships should have affiliated teams to identify promising technologies, optimize them for the field (e.g., identify adjuvants that enhance vaccine products on a small scale, to provide directionality in what to do during a surge), and consider investments required to reach efficiency yields. These partnerships should support Phase I–III clinical trials, as recommended by the United Kingdom/G7 Independent Panel for Pandemic Preparedness and Response, as well as early dosing trials. They should also build in workforce development

training for areas of expertise required to be "at the table" for technology transfer of these products.

d. Government–industry partnerships should share workforce development requirements with CEPI, the World Health Organization, and other relevant multilateral partners, to help countries identify and fill gaps in ministries of health, labor, and economics expertise before a pandemic.

5: An Influenza Vaccine Moonshot: Financing for Transformational Universal Influenza Vaccine R&D, Licensure, and Procurement

Universal influenza vaccines would be a complete game changer for pandemic preparedness and seasonal influenza vaccine markets. However, this is a science and not an engineering problem, these vaccines are a long shot, and there is no guarantee that any amount of money invested would yield a product broadly effective across all current and future influenza strains and provide long-term protection in people of all age groups. Universal vaccines are a problem that must be solved independently for each set of pathogens. Yet, as Harris (2021) argued, even "failed" attempts at vaccine production—such as for HIV—often generate scientific findings that can revolutionize vaccines for other diseases. This reinforces the principle of multidisciplinary problem solving. The platform technologies used for COVID-19 are arguably descendants of successful vaccines developed for Ebola, MERS, SARS-CoV-1, and human papillomavirus, and mRNA technology is being applied to new fields, such as vascular and cardiac regeneration (AstraZeneca, 2021) and immuno-oncology (personalized cancer vaccines).

Influenza poses such a high pandemic risk that, even with just a 20 percent chance of developing a successful universal vaccine, it is still worth investing billions. Such activities have not been dedicated funding proportional to their potential benefits, for both influenza and developing technologies that may be relevant for other pathogens. Transformational changes for influenza vaccine technologies will require new actors to push forward fundamental and applied research, coupled with substantive new sources of funding. While "moonshot" may be seen as a cliché, it is a useful shorthand for describing a massive concerted effort to achieve a specific, ambitious goal that has not received the requisite global resources.

Summary of findings: For influenza and other pathogens with pandemic potential, industry is often insufficiently certain of the government interests and regulatory pathway to bring a profitable product to the market. Solving a limited number of science problems for influenza and demonstrating a commercial pathway is essential to drive the broad and durable changes necessary for influenza vaccines. The Sabin-Aspen Vaccine Science and Policy Group, acknowledging that influenza was outside of CEPI's scope, called for establishing an entity dedicated to universal influenza vaccine development, which would embrace the need for innovation to invigorate the influenza vaccine landscape in 2018, and the Bill & Melinda Gates Foundation (BMGF) launched a $12 million "Ending the Pandemic Threat" Grand Challenge for universal influenza vaccine development that year. More recently, the Center for Infectious Disease Research and Policy (CIDRAP) Influenza Vaccine Road Map called for exploring the feasibility of a "mission-driven" R&D public–private partnership for universal influenza vaccines, with robust funding. It underscores the importance of working with industry to derisk vaccine R&D and develop a market for producing improved or universal influenza vaccines.

The scale of investment in universal influenza vaccines to date (millions) is nowhere near that required (billions) to incentivize the risky undertaking of universal influenza vaccine R&D. Both push and pull incentives will be critical to demonstrate a proof of concept for the market of influenza vaccines. A massive push will be required to elicit pre-competitive scientific and biological analyses for vaccine targets. CEPI's mission (CEPI, 2021a) is to "stimulate and accelerate the development of vaccines against emerging infectious diseases and enable access to these vaccines for people during outbreaks," based on an understanding that the market potential for these vaccines is limited. An expanded mandate for CEPI may allow it to lead a universal influenza vaccine push structure—which has suffered a challenging market potential—on a global, multilateral scale, if supported by sufficient funding.

Push incentives could be complemented by large-scale pull incentives. AMCs have most commonly been used by HIC donors to incentivize production and capacity for proven vaccine approaches, rather than to drive new science. For example, the G7 and BMGF committed to buy a new vaccine against LMIC-specific strains of pneumococcal disease, which Gavi is now using to vaccinate children in numerous developing countries (BMGF, n.d.). Finally, and most importantly, the world can obtain early and equitable access to priority lifesaving vaccines with assurances of sustainable and affordable supply in the future. Kremer and Glennerster (2004) originally proposed the AMC to encourage research on vaccines against technologically distant targets such as malaria; the instrument can be usefully deployed as an incentive to solve hard biology problems, such as those implicit in a universal influenza vaccine.

Conclusion 5A. *A concerted effort is needed to demonstrate the direction that pharmaceutical companies should be moving in within the influenza space, toward transformational next-generation technologies and universal influenza vaccine targets. A moonshot for a universal* *influenza vaccine, consisting of push and pull incentives, should be initiated. Acknowledging current global inequities of vaccine availability, both should include equitable access provisions.*

Conclusion 5B. *Like influenza, SARS-CoV-2 and other pandemic viruses and their variants may linger on as "seasonal" pathogens in the future, and vaccine capacity should therefore anticipate vaccine needs beyond the acute phase of a pandemic and provide incentives for their production.*

Conclusion 5C. *The influenza moonshot should include a similar quest for more broadly protective ("variant-proof") vaccines against coronaviruses with pandemic potential.*

Recommendation 5: The Global Health Threats Board or similar governance structure created by the G7/G20 pandemic preparedness and response agenda, working with other relevant organizations, should initiate a dedicated "moonshot" program to incentivize development, licensure, and eventual procurement of a universal influenza vaccine candidate as a matter of priority. This program's structure and funding should include (1) a push element for universal influenza vaccine research and development, which could be led by a variety of entities, including the Coalition for Epidemic Preparedness Innovations with input from its Scientific Advisory Committee, the Biomedical Advanced Research and Development Authority, the HERA Incubator, the World Health Organization, the U.S. Centers for Disease Control and Prevention, or other agencies that operate beyond the vaccine exploratory science phase and have a stake in market shaping, and (2) a complementary pull element (an advance market commitment [AMC]) to ensure procurement of resultant universal influenza vaccines, with technical leadership from Gavi and the United Nations Children's Fund (as a procurement agency for Gavi). This influenza moonshot should be coupled with a parallel effort for coronaviruses or other respiratory viruses with pandemic potential that produce variants of concern. Financing for the push and pull elements for both virus families should

a. Receive funding from multilateral actors, development banks, philanthropies (e.g., the Wellcome Trust and the Bill & Melinda Gates Foundation), and regional governance structures, including but not limited to the Organisation for Economic Co-operation and Development, G20, World Bank/International Monetary Fund, regional development banks, the World Trade

Organization, European Union, and African Union. This funding should be separately and individually supported by trade and global financing institutions of the United States, China, and the European Union, such as the European Investment Bank and Asian Infrastructure Investment Bank.

b. Include participation from middle-income countries (MICs). The price for participation for these countries should be value-based and tiered; it should be determined by a value assessment (e.g., Health Technology Assessment) as part of the AMC. A financial intermediary such as a multilateral development bank should underwrite MICs' own value-based AMCs, so countries do not need to put aside scarce resources until an effective product is approved.
c. Include country-specific tiered prices for guaranteed volumes of vaccines to multiple developers that meet the minimum efficacy threshold, to provide an incentive to retain multiple potential innovators. This would hedge risk against late failure of one or more early candidates and protect against the possibility of safety risks after widespread deployments that require restricted use or result in the first entrant's withdrawal from the market.
d. Include a requirement for successful vaccine innovator(s) to license their vaccines to other suppliers or manufacturers at low or zero cost, as a condition of accessing this guaranteed market. This will help facilitate widespread scale-up across all countries.
e. Be carefully costed over the next 1–2 years, to determine the scale of funding for this moonshot that could reasonably derisk investments in influenza vaccine technologies.

6: Supporting Geographically Distributed Hubs for Influenza Vaccine Manufacturing and Supply Chain Capacity

Regional hubs offer promise in countering vaccine nationalism and promoting equitable access through self-sufficiency. However, distributing manufacturing does not offer a full solution for addressing issues of vaccine equity. It has historically sometimes led to lower-quality products or provided incentives for elevated prices, such as for antiretrovirals. During the COVID-19 pandemic, nearly all vaccine candidates, with the exception of Pfizer's, were push funded, but this resulted in a major market failure in terms of access, with many low-income countries receiving just 2 percent coverage as of June 2021. As seen during the COVID-19 pandemic, vaccine nationalism may also persist *within* regions during times of scarcity, even when regional organizations, such as the AU, call for solidarity.

It is most productive to think of balancing the scale of production and regional diversification as complementary "belts and suspenders." Increasing scale does not directly address principles of equity but can help prevent vaccine hoarding. Conversely, regional diversification keeps countries more engaged, but the redundancy it creates does not guarantee that all countries in each region will benefit (and may, in fact, merely promote distributed vaccine nationalism). When designing regional hubs, care must be taken to not over-diversify or assume that—unless every continent has capacity for influenza and other vaccine production—a continent cannot be guaranteed to get supplies. Indeed, it may be better to use the label "geographically distributed manufacturing hubs" rather than "regional hubs," to avoid a presupposition that facilities must be distributed precisely by WHO regions.

Such geographically distributed manufacturing hubs are the best direction, but the precise balance of scale and diversification may ultimately depend on the vaccine technologies that emerge. Care must be taken not to advocate for a norm in which areas without regional capacity do not get served during a pandemic. As it is difficult to predict the optimal platform for each pathogen with pandemic potential, it is important to strive for diversification in terms of the number of facilities, their locations, and the types of platforms they can manufacture.

Summary of findings: As underscored by WHO's Global Action Plan (GAP) for influenza vaccines and recent WHO and International Federation of Pharmaceutical Manufacturers & Associations (IFPMA) surveys (see Chapter 4), the current influenza vaccine manufacturing capacity would be insufficient to vaccinate the world during a pandemic, even over 12 months. New technologies may compress this time line, but capacity would still need to be expanded at least 3-fold to avoid shortages fueling vaccine nationalism.

Regionally distributed manufacturing hubs are a way to provide this scaled-up vaccine manufacturing in LMICs. However, they face several challenges. First, to be sustainable, they must have both government commitment and strong industry involvement. Second, to be successful, particularly in geographic areas that currently lack manufacturing capacity for mRNA and other platform technologies (e.g., Africa), new facilities and partnerships will require a strong business model. This has traditionally been problematic for influenza because vaccines have had poor local and regional markets, due in large part to egg-based vaccines' low efficacy and lack of national vaccination plans. Platform technologies may provide a solution, but only if hubs can keep their facilities "warm" (actively producing vaccines or other products) between pandemics. Third, to have the capacity to develop a product that can be licensed and exported, they require workforce training for technology transfer and regulatory capacity. This is a largely unregulated field; while CEPI recently launched a survey with governments (CEPI, 2021b) to map the landscape of vaccine manufacturing capacity and capability in Africa, Southeast Asia, the Middle East, and Latin America, regional manufacturers have struggled to know what other manufacturers are working on and where they may obtain relevant technical advice and training. Fourth, to be successful, a business model must further include provision for developing plans for who will get vaccines, where, and how. Keeping national plans updated is the biggest challenge for developing regional capacity (every country must be willing and able to receive a vaccine, if it is made at a hub outside of its borders).

The GAP program focused on egg-based technologies, and any future global partnerships for diversified manufacturing and supply chain coordination should be designed to sustain newer technologies and provide long-term demand certainties. Manufacturers deeply entrenched in seasonal influenza have a residual commitment to argue that it needs to retain separate capacity. Increasing seasonal influenza vaccine demand as a principle for expanding global manufacturing (WHO, 2021b) capacity remains important—but current demands for seasonal production are not sufficient to support expansion to meet the demands during a pandemic. A business model for pandemic influenza vaccines requires a business plan for manufacturing facilities to keep them functioning between pandemics. In addition to seasonal influenza, assuming that platforms are appropriate, vaccines could be produced during times of no disease pandemics for other regional priority pathogens, such as MERS (which has a relatively small market but would be an "easy" target for applying coronavirus platform technologies), Zika, Ebola, and dengue or, if applicable, current vaccine-preventable diseases that require routine immunization (e.g., polio).

Market shaping and procurement for these products, such as Gavi's activities for pneumococcal vaccines, is critical. This downstream market issue is different from upstream technology and R&D issues and not specific to influenza. However, no global institutional architecture exists to handle this issue, and development finance institutions often struggle to develop business cases for vaccines for a pandemic with uncertain timing. During COVID-19, CEPI performed early manufacturing scale-up, and BARDA supported scale-up through OWS, but this manufacturing support was provided *after* the pandemic began. In April 2021, WHO issued a global call for "expression of interest" in establishing COVID-19 mRNA vaccine technology transfer hubs, which could scale up production and access to COVID-19 vaccines. In partnership with COVID-19 Vaccines Global Access (COVAX), the Africa CDC, a network of universities, and an industry consortium (Biovac, Afrigen Biologics and Vaccines), the first COVID-19 mRNA vaccine technology transfer hub is planned for South Africa (WHO, 2021c). This is a crucial step in building geographically distributed manufacturing hub capacity, but additional investments will be necessary on a much larger scale.

Furthermore, one cannot think about distribution and redundancy in terms of manufacturing and regulation alone. During COVID-19, supply chains broke down, and these have often been the reason that we could not produce more vaccines faster. Geographical distribution is about not only having factories and research facilities but also ensuring that these factories have key inputs that they need to produce vaccines and the flexibility to diversify their production. Developing geographically distributed supply chain hubs in parallel to manufacturing facilities presents a market opportunity for countries to invest as suppliers in the bags, filters, and other items required for vaccine supply chains. Supply chains are complicated by the fact that decisions about requirements (bioreactor bags, etc.) are made at the company level, such that pieces are often not interoperable or standardized between companies and may not meet the distribution capabilities of LMICs. Changes will not be enacted unless they have an umbrella that protects industry, but changes are required because current supply chains represent a bottleneck for vaccine scale-up. Supply chains are often treated like they are just something you need for manufacturing, but being a supplier is also a business.

CEPI has provided support for the geographically distributed hub realm in three major ways, in the capacity of a "utility infielder" or catalyst. First, it has looked for bilateral arrangements between specific and willing partners and considered how they can be supported to facilitate technology transfer (e.g., facilitating a licensing agreement between AstraZeneca and the Serum Institute of India for COVID-19 vaccine supplies for LMICs). Second, it has provided technical support to regional efforts for capacity building, for example through a memorandum of understanding with the AU during COVID-19 (CEPI, 2021d). Third, it has worked with development banks to provide technical support to LMICs and other clients for developing funding proposals (CEPI, 2020), in the context of distributed vaccine manufacturing.

Conclusion 6A. *Scaling up production of pandemic influenza vaccines requires investment in manufacturing, which may be best accomplished through technological assistance for and investments in geographically distributed hubs—facilities that can produce platform technologies both for evolving influenza vaccines and other targets. Supply chain commodity production requires similar attributes to vaccine production.*

Conclusion 6B. *Developing an ecosystem for geographically distributed manufacturing hubs requires holistic consideration of the requirements for sustainability and success, including technology transfer and workforce development for platform technologies; regulatory capacity* *to produce vaccines; and a business model that creates a market for products developed using platform technologies (with the ability to rapidly switch to pandemic production mode) during times of no disease pandemics. A sustainable business model should address the "demand" (see Recommendation 7) for the products developed, such as their ability to be introduced into national or other immunization programs (including the burden of illness and appetite), and account for how new vaccines may need to be scaled up at different times of year (not traditional influenza seasons) and at different intervals. This requires actively considering new technologies coming onto the market and tying them to industry strategies and partnerships with appropriate manufacturing facilities.*

Conclusion 6C. *Like manufacturing, geographically distributed supply chains should be coordinated, dual use, and interoperable, backed by a sustainable business model and redundancy. Forming geographically distributed manufacturing and supply chain hubs, which are capable of scaling up platform technologies in the context of a pandemic and in environments currently underserved by technology, will require sustained international investment and technical training. This training should include long-term, targeted workforce development, under the auspices of a plan to transition to local ownership and staffing.*

Recommendation 6: The Global Health Threats Board or similar governance structure created by the G7/G20 pandemic preparedness response agenda should initiate a *long-term* (10–20+ years) multilateral partnership to track emerging technologies that may be targets for technology transfer for vaccines for influenza; promote industry partnerships with geographically distributed hubs; and provide technical training. To do so, it should do the following:

a. Identify or create an international entity to assume responsibility for catalyzing voluntary technology transfer initiatives for platform technologies, including influenza vaccines. The structure's governance should build on both the World Health Organization's and COVAX's work on the COVID-19 mRNA hub, expanding it to include a diverse portfolio of technologies capable of providing protection against diverse threats with pandemic potential, and the COVAX Vaccine Manufacturing Taskforce, expanding it to work with vaccine manufacturing bodies to identify supply chain inputs and needs across a variety of vaccine candidates.
b. Ensure that this entity promotes the development of platforms suited to the production of vaccines for other pathogens of national or regional importance in addition to seasonal in-

fluenza—or products such as therapeutics—including tracking technologies coming onto the market and building platforms for voluntary industry collaboration.

c. **Develop or assist with the development of plans for geographically distributed hub training requirements, such as vaccine regulatory needs and vaccine product sourcing.**
d. **Encourage countries considering warming their manufacturing capacity for influenza vaccines and vaccines for other pathogens with pandemic potential to consider whether their focus should instead be on building new production capacity of key manufacturing inputs for vaccine manufacturing.**
e. **Be given dedicated funding to support these activities from the World Bank and regional development banks, in conjunction with the International Finance Corporation.**

7: Last Mile to the Goal of Vaccination: Generating Influenza Vaccine Demand Through Globally Coordinated Deployment Activities

Vaccines do not save lives, vaccination saves lives. Deployment capability does not automatically exist just because many vaccines are available. Even in countries such as the United States, the COVID-19 pandemic has demonstrated how vaccine availability and success at achieving high vaccination rates are different issues and present serious challenges. Experiences with the ACT Accelerator show how multilateral actors and governments alike consistently underestimated the challenges at the deployment end of the vaccination chain. Countries therefore need to build and sustain deployment capability. This is particularly necessary because deployment is not just about the public health benefits of getting vaccines into arms; demand can also have a "warming" or "chilling" effect on vaccine markets. Scaling up delivery capacity quickly can also provide a window where people are very motivated because the disease is at its highest prevalence. This creates a strong financial sustainability market, particularly for upcoming geographically distributed manufacturing facilities, to invest in national plans and infrastructure for deployment.

Summary of findings: Vaccine financing programs often focus more on procurement than the programmatic needs to ensure that vaccines become vaccinations. Many countries, particularly LMICs, lack adult vaccine deployment plans and experience, including for seasonal and pandemic influenza. Deployment activities require proper technical guidance and designated financial resources, but care should be taken not to frame deployment as a positive externality. UNICEF and Gavi have decades-long experience in deployment planning, implementation, supply chains, monitoring, and policies. Both are well positioned to take the lead on global coordination for vaccine deployment, particularly in LMICs. Large nongovernmental organizations (NGOs) active in the field, such as the Bangladesh Rural Advancement Committee in Bangladesh, can also play a crucial role in engagement and vaccine confidence at the local community level. WHO has expertise in providing technical guidance on national pandemic and vaccination planning and country readiness assessments, including reaching high-risk populations.

Conclusion 7A. *A vaccine market supported by an immunization program able to deliver vaccines coupled with a population demand for these vaccines are essential elements to ensure a sustainable vaccine manufacturing base. Stronger national plans for deployment of seasonal influenza vaccines (using next-generation/platform technologies) and recognizing that vaccines will increasingly be available across the human lifespan (WHO, 2021d) are essential factors for vaccine markets and have a strong public health rationale. Gavi, UNICEF, and WHO can facilitate national and regional coordination for deployment activities.*

Recommendation 7: The United Nations Children's Fund, Gavi, and relevant national and regional organizations (including governments) should be given funding explicitly allocated for introducing and deploying next-generation seasonal influenza vaccines to underpin scaled-up manufacturing capacity. The World Health Organization regional offices should urgently work with countries to do more extensive assessments of their readiness to reach appropriate populations, including adults and high-risk groups, to enable work plans by 2023, which include the following:

a. An analysis of what infrastructure (e.g., data and digitization of immunization records) built for COVID can be adapted, strengthened, and sustained for at least one additional adult and one adolescent vaccine.
b. Advising member states on best practices used in countries that had high immunization rates during COVID-19.
c. Assisting member states to look at their data and logistics systems for monitoring coverage and for tracking safety (pharmacovigilance) and on the options for adopting no-fault compensation as part of patient safety mechanisms.

THE PATH FORWARD

In a historically unprecedented way, security for people around the world now depends on global cooperation. Acting and investing collectively for

> pandemic security, together with climate change, represents the primary international challenge of our times. Failure to establish the basis for international cooperation will make it almost impossible to address these existential challenges. (HLIP, 2021)

In its deliberations, the Committee on Global Coordination, Partnerships, and Financing Recommendations for Advancing Pandemic and Seasonal Influenza Vaccine Preparedness and Response arrived at a set of views similar to those of the G20 HLIP, although these had not yet been released yet. The terms "coordination," "partnerships," and "financing" in the committee's title represent three key areas on which our future ability to protect the global human population from catastrophic pandemics depend. It is the committee's hope that its messages on the crucial need to improve progress in each of these three areas are clear.

This study was completed in a much shorter time than is allowed for typical National Academies consensus studies, with only 5 months for both deliberations and report drafting. The Statement of Task was also very broad and asked the committee to reflect on lessons learned for governance and financing from the COVID-19 pandemic response—which is itself still in active motion. Most of the committee's deliberations took place before critical reports from the PPR agenda were released, particularly the G20's HLIP. Furthermore, many additional PPR-related reports from the G7, G20 and many other actors—as well as the WHA's discussions on a potential pandemic treaty or instrument—are upcoming in late 2021 and 2022.

In this context, the committee fully acknowledges that it was unable to delve deeply into many relevant topics, and some of its recommendations lack specificity in actors. The latter imprecision is necessary and deliberate; it enables the recommendations to, as much as possible, be aligned with the evolving global infrastructural architecture and roles designed in real time by the G7 and G20's PPR agendas. We hope that one of the principal tasks of the G7 and G20 will be to identify more specific actors, institutional arrangements, and financing mechanisms for pandemic threats—including influenza—to ensure accountability and provide necessary resources. A first task of the emergent Global Health Threats Board (or the entity designed with this mandate) should be to develop a pathway for providing this level of specificity.

The committee explicitly devised its recommendations on the assumption that the G7 and G20 will pursue a coordinated approach to PPR, with a governance mechanism and potentially a new international pandemic governance instrument. However, the committee recognizes that this assumption is not a forgone conclusion, despite the compelling economic and human case for collective action to reinforce PPR. Because international coordination mechanisms, including a pandemic treaty or special international instrument, may not withstand nationalistic impulses that such an agreement inevitably generates, it is all the more important to minimize dependence on such mechanisms. This underscores the importance of (1) advancing vaccine science as much as possible, (2) building as much manufacturing scale as possible, and (3) identifying the components of the influenza and PPR system that can be made neutral or resilient to national pressures.

The changing dynamics of international relations over the last decade or so have transformed the geopolitical context in which global health policy is made. Shifts in the balance of power in the international system, the rise of authoritarian states, diminished cohesion of democratic states, and the rise of nationalism and populism across a broad array of states are among the factors that have led to this transformation. The COVID-19 response exposed sharp fissures in the international order, shaking confidence in the notion of a "global community" and revealing the powerful, complex, and somewhat contradictory interactions between global health priorities, domestic political imperatives, and other dimensions of geopolitical competition and collaboration. Major powers in the G7 and G20 have simultaneously supported efforts to promote equitable access to vaccines and actively engaged in "vaccine nationalism." Meanwhile "vaccine diplomacy" has been used to garner geopolitical and ideological advantage. One of the biggest and most sobering lessons from COVID-19 is that in an infectious disease crisis of this magnitude, neither established arrangements, such as the International Health Regulations, nor newly created mechanisms, such as COVAX, can withstand the overwhelming pressures to prioritize national interests.

The committee did not directly consider how to address these daunting geopolitical challenges, as doing so would have involved venturing far beyond its mandate. However, the committee recognizes that overcoming these challenges, or at least mitigating their consequences for global health, is a prerequisite for success for both the PPR agenda and the specific influenza vaccine recommendations that this committee put forward. That a geopolitical context can be established in which one can speak meaningfully of a "global community" able to take at least some degree of coordinated collective action is, in a sense, a basic assumption that the committee adopted, since much of what is proposed in the recommendations requires this as a foundation. This does not require global consensus on everything or mean that every country is involved in every effort, but it implies a base level of coordination among leading states. As a shorthand expression and recognizing that this is an imperfect depiction of the stakeholders involved, this report typically refers to the G7 and G20 as the nexus of such a global community.

The committee also recognizes that there may be scope to construct some technical coordination mechanisms in more of a "flying under the radar" mode and thus somewhat insulated from politics. However, the committee is skeptical about relying too much on such an approach. COVID-19 has repeatedly revealed how the intense political pressures that arise from a deadly pandemic can override technical, contractual, or legal considerations. As the G7 and G20 devise a new set of arrangements for PPR, including potential legal obligations (e.g., from a pandemic treaty or instrument, should such emerge), governance mechanisms (such as a Global Health Threats Board), and financing programs (such as HLIP's proposed Global Health Threats Fund), it is important to recognize that when put to the test, these new arrangements are unlikely to work as precisely as designed. Once again, national interests will prove almost impossible to withstand. But recognizing their limitations does not equate to believing that such arrangements have no value: they can be enormously helpful in shifting norms and behaviors, such as toward more equitable deployment of lifesaving medical tools.

The committee wishes to highlight several critical areas that are essential for refinement of the PPR agenda and either fell outside of the Statement of Task or were unable to be fully analyzed within the study's time frame. We list them below, view them as having equal levels of priority, and recommend that all be more fully addressed or explored over the next 2–3 years.

First, the term "sustainability" is often used and considered narrowly, rather than holistically. Sustainability is inseparable from a number of uncertainties about the future and global trends, which means that the next major epidemic or pandemic may look very different from COVID-19. For example, an influenza pandemic could be milder or more severe in terms of transmissibility and lethality and could be regional or global. Rapid urbanization patterns and global warming may also change the types and trajectories of emerging infectious diseases. This uncertain landscape must be considered when designing "sustainable" influenza and respiratory PPR initiatives for the future. One clearly visible trend amid this uncertainty is vaccine confidence. COVID-19 has changed the way that the world—and public health professionals—view vaccine confidence and hesitancy. Uptake of available vaccines is likely to be even lower in the context of the "known" threat of influenza, where vaccines have often had low efficacy. Much more work should be done on pre-pandemic communication strategies and national planning that could improve vaccine confidence across diseases and lead to increased recognition of the dangers of influenza among members of the public. This will require careful country surveys and risk assessments, which extend beyond the capacity of this study. Phenomena such as the current vaccine hesitancy in the United States would appear to be partly the result of politicization but could occur elsewhere under other circumstances.

Second, there has been frequent "hand-waving" about the importance of One Health. What remains blurry is how the coordination between animal and human health can be made more effective and efficient. One Health accomplishments have been mostly based on rhetoric or goodwill between specific individuals working at particular organizations rather than a truly effective set of processes. The World Organisation for Animal Health, the Food and Agriculture Organization of the United Nations, WHO, and the United Nations Environment Programme are all critical actors in developing such processes, and these institutions have seen some recent momentum for One Health, such as a recent announcement about the establishment of an expert panel (WHO, 2021e) comprising representatives from these four agencies and designed to strengthen and deepen their cooperation around the emergence and spread of zoonotic diseases. Much more work is needed to align objectives across these institutions in the context of pandemic threats and back these objectives with dedicated financial resources. We mostly considered this realm from the perspective of surveillance financing for influenza and respiratory pathogens with pandemic potential, but this funding is best seen as the tip of the iceberg in terms of the One Health collaboration required for zoonotic disease PPR. Even the current debate and terminology of PPR understates the importance of prevention, particularly pre-spillover prevention.

Third, a pandemic "treaty," if well designed, could provide a good opportunity to move from rhetoric to multilateral action on One Health for influenza and other respiratory pathogens with pandemic potential. This "treaty" could go in multiple directions, and we have endorsed principles that should be used as its foundations—but not a particular pathway for its negotiation. A convention (along the lines of the FCTC) agreement, or other framework pathway, could be pursued. Treaties or other pathways can exist between as few as two countries. Binding commitments or conventions for global access and countermeasure development programs are also good examples of agreements that might not involve a high percentage of the world's countries. The FCTC is an example of a truly global treaty, but the G7 and G20 together would also cover a significant portion of the world population if they were involved exclusively in a treaty, convention, or other framework for pandemic preparedness. How a treaty (or alternative framework) is negotiated—and whether most LMICs and HICs sign on to it—will have major implications for how the world conceptualizes pandemic threats. Wide sign-on by the United States, China, and a high number of LMICs and HICs will be necessary for this treaty or framework to embrace pandemic preparedness as a global public good, rather than merely an issue of global security. Careful consideration of the PIP Framework's core principles and the aforementioned "grand bargain" will be essential for successful negotiations.

Fourth, ambiguity remains about the right size for a sustainable vaccine market that would allow for a sufficient surge during an influenza pandemic.

Particularly with the possibility for "platform-agnostic" production with next-generation vaccines (i.e., the ability for geographically distributed hubs or central manufacturers to produce mRNA or recombinant vaccines, beyond seasonal influenza, during times of no disease pandemics), it will be critical to consider how to balance obsolete capacity between pandemics and the need for surge potential when a pandemic strikes. This will require in-depth market analyses, with careful consideration of pricing pressures and business response. Such an analysis will be instrumental in allowing the proposed global manufacturing hub coordination actor (e.g., CEPI) to develop plans that balance the inefficiencies of having multiple small, distributed manufacturing facilities with the cost efficiencies of centralized manufacturing facilities. Unfortunately, this important analysis extended beyond the resources and time allotted for this study.

Lastly, more work should be done to determine the size of public subsidy that would be required to sustain this specific level of manufacturing capacity and the magnitude of public funding that would be required to meaningfully move forward with a universal influenza moonshot. This costing will be critical for priority-setting for influenza in the PPR agenda.

We hope that by advancing a global public goods framework for influenza, which links—and prioritizes—it with other respiratory viral diseases with pandemic potential, influenza will be recognized as a serious pandemic threat and afforded funding commensurate with its economic and public health risks. It will be critical for HICs and middle-income countries to extend their resource allocation for PPR. In advancing this framework, we recognize the principles of equity and human rights, which have not been fully embraced by global coordination mechanisms during COVID-19. At the same time, we underscore that it is critical to remember that obligations attached to industry through partnerships or ABS will determine how industry reacts—and both transformative R&D and sustainable vaccine markets are unlikely to emerge without strong industry support. The path forward for global influenza PPR will require engagement of and coordination among diverse actors, spanning civil society, industry, national entities, bilateral organizations, and multilateral organizations. Each actor will need to recognize the need to temper self-interest to counter the pandemic threat and address the *influenza imperative*.

REFERENCES

AstraZeneca. 2021. *Entering a new era in vascular and cardiac regeneration research*. https://www.astrazeneca.com/what-science-can-do/topics/next-generation-therapeutics/entering-a-new-era-in-vascular-and-cardiac-regeneration-research.html (accessed August 12, 2021).

BMGF (Bill & Melinda Gates Foundation). n.d. Kenya marks the global roll-out of pneumococcal vaccine. https://www.gatesfoundation.org/ideas/media-center/press-releases/2011/02/kenya-marks-the-global-rollout-of-pneumococcal-vaccine (accessed December 19, 2021).

CEPI (Coalition for Epidemic Preparedness Innovations). 2020. *Call for proposals: Achieving an unprecedented acceleration of vaccine development and global manufacturing capacity to prevent COVID-19*. https://cepi.net/wp-content/uploads/2020/05/Call-text_COVID-19_CFP-2C_04052020_website.pdf (accessed August 12, 2021).

CEPI. 2021a. *Our mission: New vaccines for a safer world*. https://cepi.net/about/whyweexist (accessed August 12, 2021).

CEPI. 2021b. *Survey launched by CEPI to track multinational vaccine manufacturing capacity for use in future epidemics and pandemics*. https://cepi.net/news_cepi/survey-launched-by-cepi-to-track-multinational-vaccine-manufacturing-capacity-for-use-in-future-epidemics-and-pandemics (accessed August 12, 2021).

CEPI. 2021c. *CEPI and the African Union join forces to boost African vaccine R&D and manufacturing*. https://cepi.net/news_cepi/cepi-and-the-african-union-join-forces-to-boost-african-vaccine-rd-and-manufacturing (accessed August 12, 2021).

Harris, J. E. 2021. *The repeated setbacks of HIV vaccine development laid the groundwork for Sars-Cov-2 vaccines*. Working Paper 28587. Cambridge, MA: National Bureau of Economic Research. http://www.nber.org/papers/w28587 (accessed August 12, 2021).

HLIP (High-Level Independent Panel). 2021. *A global deal for our pandemic age: Report of the G20 High-Level Independent Panel on Financing the Global Commons for Pandemic Preparedness and Response*. https://pandemic-financing.org/report/foreword (accessed October 24, 2021).

Kremer, M., and R. Glennerster. 2004. *Strong nedicine: Creating incentives for pharmaceutical research on neglected diseases*. Princeton, NJ: Princeton University Press.

The Rockefeller Foundation. 2021. *The Rockefeller Foundation announces key grants and collaborations to strengthen global genomic sequencing and data sharing*. Press release 06/09/2021. https://www.rockefellerfoundation.org/news/the-rockefeller-foundation-announces-key-grants-and-collaborations-toward-the-creation-of-a-pandemic-prevention-institute (accessed August 12, 2021).

Sabin-Aspen Vaccine Science and Policy Group. 2019. *Accelerating the development of a universal influenza vaccine: A report from the Sabin-Aspen Vaccine Science and Policy Group*. https://www.influenzer.org/app/uploads/2020/01/sabin-aspen-report-digital.pdf (accessed August 12, 2021).

West African Health Organization. n.d. *The Regional Disease Surveillance Systems Enhancement (REDISSE) Project in West Africa*. https://www.wahooas.org/web-ooas/en/projets/redisse-regional-disease-surveillance-systems-enhancement-project-west-africa (accessed August 12, 2021).

WHO (World Health Organization). 2021a. *The public health implications of implementation of the Nagoya Protocol: Report by the WHO Director-General*. EB148/21. https://apps.who.int/gb/ebwha/pdf_files/EB148/B148_21-en.pdf (accessed August 12, 2021).

WHO. 2021b. *Global Action Plan for Influenza Vaccines: FAQ*. https://www.who.int/influenza_vaccines_plan/resources/gap_faq.pdf?ua=1 (accessed August 12, 2021).

WHO. 2021c. *WHO supporting South African consortium to establish first COVID mRNA vaccine technology transfer hub*. News release, June 21, 2021. https://www.who.int/news/item/21-06-2021-who-supporting-south-african-consortium-to-establish-first-covid-mrna-vaccine-technology-transfer-hub (accessed August 12, 2021).

WHO. 2021d. *Immunization Agenda 2030: A global strategy to leave no one behind*. https://www.who.int/teams/immunization-vaccines-and-biologicals/strategies/ia2030 (accessed December 19, 2021).

WHO. 2021e. *New international expert panel to address the emergence and spread of zoonotic diseases*. https://www.who.int/news/item/20-05-2021-new-international-expert-panel-to-address-the-emergence-and-spread-of-zoonotic-diseases (accessed August 12, 2021).

Yamey, G., M. Schäferhoff, M. Pate, M. Chawla, K. Ranson, F. Zhao, R. Hatchett, and R. Wilder. 2020. *Funding the development and manufacturing of COVID-19 vaccines*. Duke Global Working Paper 20. https://papers.ssrn.com/sol3/papers.cfm?abstract_id=3575660 (accessed August 12, 2021).

Appendix A

Committee and Staff Biographies

Peter Sands, M.P.A. (*Chair*), has been the executive director of The Global Fund to Fight AIDS, Tuberculosis and Malaria since March 2018. Since June 2015, he has been a research fellow at Harvard University, dividing his time between the Mossavar-Rahmani Center for Business and Government at the Harvard Kennedy School and the Harvard Global Health Institute. Mr. Sands was the group chief executive officer of Standard Chartered PLC from November 2006 to June 2015, having joined the board of Standard Chartered as group chief financial officer in May 2002. Earlier, he was a senior partner at McKinsey & Company. Mr. Sands graduated from Oxford University with a first-class degree in politics, philosophy, and economics. He also received an M.P.A. from Harvard University, where he was a Harkness Fellow. Mr. Sands has served on various boards and commissions, including the UK Department of Health, the World Economic Forum, and the International Advisory Board of the Monetary Authority of Singapore. In 2016–2017, he chaired the International Working Group on Financing Pandemic Preparedness at the World Bank. In 2015–2016, he was the chair of the U.S. National Academy of Medicine's Commission on a Global Health Risk Framework for the Future, which published the influential report *The Neglected Dimension of Global Security: A Framework to Counter Infectious Disease Threats* in January 2016. Mr. Sands is also a member of the National Academies' Forum on Microbial Threats and served on the Committee on Ensuring Patient Access to Affordable Drugs Therapies.

Devi Sridhar, D.Phil., M.Phil. (*Vice Chair*), is a professor at the University of Edinburgh Medical School and holds a personal chair in global public health. She is the founding director of the Global Health Governance Programme and won a Wellcome Trust Investigator Award. She was the associate professor in global health politics and a fellow at Wolfson College and a postdoctoral research fellow at All Souls College, both at Oxford University. She was also a visiting associate professor at Ludwig Maximilian University of Munich and a guest lecturer at the Harvard T.H. Chan School of Public Health and Public Health Foundation of India. Her books include *Governing Global Health: Who Runs the World and Why?* (Oxford University Press, 2017) and *The Battle Against Hunger: Choice, Circumstance and the World Bank* (Oxford University Press, 2007), and she has published in *Nature*, *Science*, *New England Journal of Medicine*, *Lancet*, and *British Medical Journal*. She served on the board of Save the Children UK and the World Economic Forum Council on the Health Industry and co-chaired the Harvard/London School of Hygiene & Tropical Medicine Independent Panel on the Global Response to Ebola. She holds a D.Phil. and an M.Phil. from Oxford University as a Rhodes Scholar and a B.S. from the University of Miami in the Honors Medical Program. Her work is concentrated in three areas: international health organizations, financing of global public health, and development of better tools for priority-setting.

Salah T. Al Awaidy, M.D., is a communicable diseases advisor in Health Affairs, Ministry of Health (MoH), Muscat, Oman. He is a medical doctor with an M.A. in epidemiology. He is the advisor on communicable disease surveillance, elimination and eradication of communicable diseases of public health importance, Expanded Program on Immunization, vaccine supply chain system, and the International Health Regulations (IHR) at the MoH, Oman. He was the director of communicable disease surveillance and control at the MoH, Oman (1997–2011), IHR national focal point (2002–2013), and a member of several of the professional committees: Strategic Advisory Group on Immunization, WHO, Geneva (2005–2007); Strategic Advisor Group on Vaccine and Store Management Training Courses (2005–2008), WHO; Strategic TB Advisory Board (2007–2011) and AIDS Regional Advisory Group, WHO Eastern Mediterranean Regional Office since 2005; and a member of the Gavi Independent Review Committee since 2014. He also serves on the IHR Emergency Committee on Polio and MERS-CoV. He was a member and the secretary of the National Immunization Technical Advisory Group of the MoH, Oman from 1997 to August 2011. Dr. Al Awaidy has been involved in research related to vaccine-preventable diseases, communicable diseases surveillance, and other communicable diseases, locally, regionally, and globally. He has played a pivotal role in national preparedness and management of SARS, pH1N1, and avian influenza; eradication of polio; elimination of measles, rubella, maternal and neonatal tetanus; leprosy; and control of tuberculosis, schistosomiasis, and other vaccine-preventable diseases. Under his leadership, Oman established a certified Central Vaccine Store and was also certified as dracunculiasis and polio free.

William Ampofo, Ph.D., is an associate professor and the head of the virology department, Noguchi Memorial Institute for Medical Research, College of Health Sciences, University of Ghana. Dr. Ampofo runs the National Influenza Center, National HIV Drug Resistance Genotyping laboratory, and serves as the laboratory focal point for the National Emergency Operations Center of the Ministry of Health. He is a member of various national bodies, including the IHR Steering Committee, HIV Technical Working Group, and Food and Drugs Authority Technical Advisory Committee on Vaccines and Biologicals. He has conducted temporary assignments throughout Africa on behalf of the World Health Organization (WHO), the Commonwealth Secretariat Health Division, the U.S. Department of Defense, the German International Development Agency, and the U.S. Agency for International Development. Since 2011, he has also served on WHO advisory groups for influenza, including global vaccine production, immunization, and pandemic preparedness. He was an advisor for the WHO IHR Emergency Committee on Ebola. Dr. Ampofo is the chair of the African Vaccine Manufacturing Initiative, the senior editor for the *African Journal for Laboratory Medicine*, and the ambassador for Ghana, African Society for Laboratory Medicine.

Phyllis Arthur, M.B.A., is responsible for working with member companies in vaccines, molecular diagnostics, and biodefense on policy, legislative, and regulatory issues in her role at the Biotechnology Innovation Association (BIO). Ms. Arthur joined BIO in July 2009 as the director of health care regulatory affairs. Earlier, she worked in numerous marketing and sales positions in Merck, Inc.'s vaccine division. Over her 16-year career in vaccines, Ms. Arthur launched several exciting new vaccines in the United States and internationally, including the first human papillomavirus vaccine, Gardasil. During her years in marketing, she worked closely with clinical and academic thought leaders in infectious diseases, oncology, and public health. In addition, Ms. Arthur also led a large vaccine sales organization of more than 75 representatives and managers covering 14 states. Before graduate school, Ms. Arthur was a research assistant for two economists at the Brookings Institution in Washington, DC, where she conducted analyses related to savings and investment policies for the Organisation for Economic Co-operation and Development countries. Ms. Arthur received her B.A. in 1987 in economics and international politics from Goucher College and her M.B.A. in 1991 from the Wharton School of Business at the University of Pennsylvania.

Christopher T. Bauch, Ph.D., is in the Department of Applied Mathematics, University of Waterloo, Canada. He specializes in the mathematical modeling of infectious diseases, the impact of interventions such as vaccines, and the applications of game theory to studying vaccine decision making. He earned his Ph.D. in mathematics from the University of Warwick in 2000. He has worked with partners such as the Bill & Melinda Gates Foundation, the World Health Organization, and the U.S. Food and Drug Administration on problems in vaccination policy. He has published more than 100 peer-reviewed journal articles, reviews, and opinion pieces on this research topic, in journals including *Science*, *Lancet Infectious Diseases*, and *Proceedings of the National Academy of Sciences of the United States of America*.

Gian Luca Burci, J.S.D., is an adjunct professor of international law at the Graduate Institute of International and Development Studies, Geneva, since 2012. Since 2016, Dr. Burci has been a visiting professor and a senior scholar at the O'Neill Center on National and Global Health Law at the Georgetown University School of Law. Before the Graduate Institute, Dr. Burci served in the World Health Organization (WHO) Legal Office from 1998 to 2016 and was its legal counsel from 2005 to 2016. Dr. Burci worked in the Department of International Cooperation of the International Atomic Energy Agency (1998–1999) and the United Nations (UN) Office of the Legal Counsel, where he was designated focal point for UN economic sanctions (1989–1998). During his service at WHO, he was involved in revising and implementing the International Health Regulations, WHO's response to the 2009–2010 H1N1 influenza pandemic and the 2014–2016 Ebola outbreak, and institutional aspects of WHO reform. Dr. Burci holds a postgraduate degree in law from the University of Genova, Italy. His areas of expertise are public international law, the law and practice of international organizations, and global health governance and law. His courses at the Graduate Institute include the law and practice of international organizations, international legal advising and advocacy, and global health law. Dr. Burci is the co-author of the leading English book on WHO, the editor of the first research collection on global health law, the co-editor of the first research handbook on global health law, and the author of numerous articles and book chapters.

Keiji Fukuda, M.D., M.P.H., is the director and a clinical professor at The University of Hong Kong School of Public Health. He worked at the World Health Organization (WHO) in Geneva as the assistant director-general for health security, the special advisor to the director-general for pandemic influenza and antimicrobial resistance, and the director of the Global Influenza Program. Before that, he worked at the U.S. Centers for

Disease Control and Prevention (CDC) as the epidemiology chief of the Influenza Branch. He has been a global public health leader in many areas. At CDC, he led the first field teams that investigated the emergence of H5N1 in Hong Kong in 1997 and worked in China on the emergence and control of the U.S. Centers for Disease Control and Prevention (CDC) in 2003 and later on the global re-emergence of H5N1. In the United States, he oversaw national influenza disease surveillance and worked on influenza vaccination guidelines and pandemic preparedness. At WHO, he supervised the Global Influenza Surveillance Network and the response to the 2009 H1N1 pandemic. He led several field missions related to the emergence and control of Middle East respiratory syndrome in Saudi Arabia and Korea, Ebola in West Africa in 2014, and H5N1 in Egypt. He was responsible for WHO's global influenza surveillance, biannual global influenza vaccine recommendations, influenza pandemic preparedness work, and oversight of the International Health Regulations and participated in global negotiations on the Pandemic Influenza Preparedness Framework, the Global Health Security Agenda, and antimicrobial resistance. He was a member of the Forum on Microbial Threats of the National Academies and currently advises the Hong Kong government on its COVID-19 response and vaccines and antimicrobial resistance. He received his B.A. from Oberlin College (1978), M.D. from the University of Vermont (1984), M.P.H. from the University of California, Berkeley (1989), and Epidemic Intelligence Service training at CDC.

Bruce G. Gellin, M.D., M.P.H., is the former president of Global Immunization at the Sabin Vaccine Institute in Washington, DC, where he oversaw Sabin's mission to make vaccines more accessible, enable innovation, and expand immunization across the globe. In June 2021, he transitioned to The Rockefeller Foundation, where he is currently the chief of global public health strategy. Dr. Gellin served at the U.S. Department of Health and Human Services (HHS) as the deputy assistant secretary for health and the director of the National Vaccine Program Office. Dr. Gellin has had broad experience in public health aspects of infectious diseases. He has held positions at the U.S. National Institutes of Health, U.S. the U.S. Centers for Disease Control and Prevention (CDC), The Rockefeller Foundation, the Vanderbilt University School of Medicine, and the Johns Hopkins Bloomberg School of Public Health. He was the founder and the executive director of the National Network for Immunization Information, intended to be a resource of up-to-date, authoritative information about vaccines and immunizations. Dr. Gellin earned a B.A. (Highest Honors) from the University of North Carolina at Chapel Hill, where he graduated Phi Beta Kappa and was a Morehead Scholar; M.D. from the Cornell University Medical College; and M.P.H. (epidemiology) from the Columbia University School of Public Health. He was a Luce Scholar in the Philippines and a Warren Weaver Fellow at The Rockefeller Foundation focused on global health. He completed his internship and residency in internal medicine at Vanderbilt University and later was a preventive medicine resident at Cornell and CDC's Arctic Investigations Program in Anchorage, Alaska, and completed a fellowship in infectious diseases at Cornell/New York Hospital. He is an adjunct professor at the Georgetown University School of Medicine with appointments in the Division of Infectious Diseases and the Center for Global Health and Security and has been a regular consultant to the World Health Organization. Among other achievements, he received the American Medical Association Nathan Davis Award, the Infectious Diseases Society of America citation for a lifetime of outstanding achievement, and HHS Secretary Award for Distinguished Service. Dr. Gellin achieved board certification in internal medicine and infectious diseases, is an active member of numerous professional organizations, serves as a peer reviewer for more than a dozen medical journals, and was a medical advisor to Encyclopedia Britannica.

Amanda L. Glassman, M.Sc., is the executive vice president and the senior fellow at the Center for Global Development (CGD) and also the chief executive officer of CGD Europe. Her research focuses on priority-setting, resource allocation, and value for money in global health, as well as data for development. She served as the director for global health policy at CGD from 2010 to 2016 and has more than 25 years of experience working on health and social protection policy and programs in Latin America and elsewhere in the developing world. Prior to joining CGD, Ms. Glassman was the principal technical lead for health at the Inter-American Development Bank, where she led policy dialogue with member countries, designed the results-based grant program Salud Mesoamerica 2015, and was the team leader for conditional cash transfer programs, such as Mexico's Oportunidades and Colombia's Familias en Accion. From 2005 to 2007, Ms. Glassman was the deputy director of the Global Health Financing Initiative at the Brookings Institution and carried out policy research on aid effectiveness and domestic financing issues in the health sector in low-income countries. Before that, she designed, supervised, and evaluated health and social protection loans at the Inter-American Development Bank and worked as a Population Reference Bureau fellow at the U.S. Agency for International Development. Ms. Glassman holds an M.Sc. from the Harvard T.H. Chan School of Public Health and a B.A. from Brown University, has published on a wide range of health and social protection finance and policy topics, and is the editor and co-author of the books *What's In, What's Out: Designing Benefits for Universal Health Coverage* (Center for Global Development, 2017), *Millions Saved: New Cases of Proven Success in Global Health* (Center for Global Development, 2016), *From Few to Many: A*

Decade of Health Insurance Expansion in Colombia (IDB and Brookings, 2010), and *The Health of Women in Latin America and the Caribbean* (World Bank, 2001).

Richard J. Hatchett, M.D., is the chief executive officer of the Coalition for Epidemic Preparedness Innovations (CEPI), a partnership of public, private, philanthropic, and civil organizations that supports vaccine development against high-priority public health threats and technology platforms to allow the rapid vaccine development against emerging infectious diseases, such as COVID-19. Dr. Hatchett was the acting director of the Biomedical Advanced Research and Development Authority and the director of medical preparedness policy on the Homeland and National Security Councils under Presidents Bush and Obama, respectively. He received his M.D. from Vanderbilt University and completed clinical training in internal medicine and medical oncology at Cornell University and Duke University.

John Nkengasong, Ph.D., M.Sc., is the director of the Africa Centres for Disease Control and Prevention. Earlier, he served as the acting deputy principal director (acting) of the Center for Global Health, U.S. Centers for Disease Control and Prevention (CDC), and chief of the International Laboratory Branch, Division of Global HIV and TB, U.S. CDC. He received an M.A. in tropical biomedical science at the Institute of Tropical Medicine in Antwerp, Belgium, and a Ph.D. in medical sciences (virology) from the University of Brussels, Belgium. He has received numerous awards for his work, including the Sheppard Award and William Watson Medal of Excellence, the highest recognition awarded by U.S. CDC. He is also recipient of the Knight of Honor Medal by the Government of Cote d'Ivoire, was knighted in 2017 as the Officer of Loin by the President of Senegal, H.E. Macky Sall, and knighted in November 2018 by the government of Cameroon for his significant contributions to public health. He is an adjunct professor at the Emory University School of Public Health. He serves on several international advisory boards, including the Coalition for Epidemic Preparedness Initiative and International AIDS Vaccine Initiative. He has authored more than 250 peer-reviewed articles in international journals and published several book chapters.

Charles "OK" Pannenborg, Ph.D., served as the World Bank's chief health scientist/director until his retirement 10 years ago, after which he was a director at Pan American Health Organization/World Health Organization (WHO), chairman of the Netherlands Commission on Global Health Research, and served on many boards in the field of global health (R&D, human resources for health, tropical diseases, biotech, etc.); he is also on the Lancet COVID-19 Commission Task Force for Global Governance. Prior to joining the World Bank in 1985, he worked for nongovernmental organizations, United Nations High Commissioner for Refugees, and WHO in several Asian and African countries, then joined the Netherlands Ministry of Health, where he directed strategic health policy, before moving to Washington, DC. During the late 1990s and 2000s, he chaired the World Bank/International Monetary Fund Pandemic Committee. He served on many technical committees of the Netherlands Medical Research Council, more recently on the National Academies of Sciences, Engineering, and Medicine's Committee on the Evaluation of Strengthening Human Resources for Health Capacity in the Republic of Rwanda under the President's Emergency Plan for AIDS Relief (PEPFAR), and he continues to advise international agencies and governments in fields of global health, such as infectious diseases, research innovation, health workforce systems, pharmaceuticals/vaccines and medical technology, and health financing and economics. Of Dr. Pannenborg's many publications, his *A New International Health Order* (1978) was among the earliest global health publications at the time.

Alexandra L. Phelan, J.S.D., LL.M., LL.B., is an assistant professor at the Center for Global Health Science and Security in the Microbiology and Immunology Department at the Georgetown University School of Medicine. She also holds an appointment as an adjunct professor of law at the Georgetown University Law Center and the Walsh School of Foreign Service. Dr. Phelan works on global public health law and governance, with a focus on emerging and reemerging infectious diseases and international law. She has worked as a consultant for the World Health Organization, the World Bank, and Gavi and advised on matters including influenza and non-influenza pathogen and genetic sequence data sharing, equitable vaccine distribution, human rights, and contract law. She is admitted to practice to the High Court of Australia and the Supreme Court of Victoria and worked as a solicitor at a large firm in Melbourne, Australia. Dr. Phelan holds an S.J.D. (2019) from the Georgetown University Law Center, where she was a General Sir John Monash Scholar. She also holds an M.S. in laws (2013), specializing in international law, from the Australian National University, a B.S. in biomedical science/laws (honors; 2009), and a diploma of languages (Mandarin Chinese; 2007) from Monash University. She is a member of the National Academies' Standing Committee on Emerging Infectious Diseases and Twenty-First Century Health Threats.

Christopher Snyder, Ph.D., has been the Joel and Susan Hyatt Professor in the Department of Economics at Dartmouth College for the past 15 years. He graduated from Fordham University with a B.A. in mathematics and economics in 1989 and received his Ph.D. in economics from the Massachusetts Institute of Technology in 1994. Dr. Snyder is a National Bureau of Economic Research research associate in the law and economics program. He is an editor for the *Journal of Law and Economics*, an associate editor for the *Review of Industrial Organization*, and the treasurer of the Industrial Organization Society. He specializes in the fields of industrial organization, law and economics, and microeconomic theory. He continues a general research interest in vertical contractual relations between firms with a recent focus on applications in health care markets. He is the co-author, with Walter Nicholson, of two widely used textbooks in intermediate microeconomics. Dr. Snyder served on expert committees that helped design the pilot advance market commitment for pneumococcus vaccine and the Global Fund's program to stockpile drugs against multidrug-resistant tuberculosis. Most recently, he advised various international and U.S. agencies on the design of the funding facilities to accelerate the development of a COVID-19 vaccine and coordinate its distribution.

Charlotte (Charlie) Weller, Ph.D., is the head of prevention at Wellcome with a focus on developing new and improved vaccines and strengthening the connection between research and decision making to ensure better use of vaccines. Her work spans multiple disease areas, including epidemics, antimicrobial resistance, and endemic diseases. Her team also manages the epidemics research work at Wellcome, which includes the Coalition for Epidemic Preparedness Innovations (CEPI). Wellcome is a founding member of CEPI and a continued funder. Dr. Weller has chaired the Investors Council since April 2020. She joined Wellcome in 2014 as a senior portfolio developer, where she oversaw the immunology portfolio, led the funding response to the Ebola epidemic of 201–2015, and contributed to strategy development in preparedness for future epidemics, prior to taking the lead on vaccines and epidemics. She has more than 16 years of research experience in both academic and pharmaceutical environments, ranging from host pathogen interactions to cellular and molecular immunology. Before joining Wellcome, she was a laboratory head at the Novartis Institute for Biomedical Research engaged in target identification and validation within the respiratory disease area, focusing on innate immune responses in respiratory exacerbations and leading multiple biologics programs. Earlier, Dr. Weller investigated mast cell localization and function in health, respiratory disease, and parasite infections as a postdoctoral fellow at Imperial College London. She holds a B.Sc. in genetics at Birmingham University and a Ph.D. in immunology at Imperial College London.

STAFF

Janelle Winters, Ph.D., M.A., M.S., was a program officer at the Board on Global Health and directed this study from its launch through entering external review. Dr. Winters is serving as a visiting assistant professor in global health studies at the University of Iowa and will take up a postdoctoral research associate post at the University of Oxford in early 2022, focused on the modern history of COVID-19 hydroxychloroquine prophylaxis trials. She holds a Ph.D. in population health sciences from the University of Edinburgh, where she was based in the Global Health Governance Group. In Edinburgh, she undertook research for the Economic Gaze project, which studied the World Bank's impact on global health. Dr. Winters has a special interest in global health partnerships and emerging infectious disease epidemiology—and the history of both. She earned an M.A. in the history of medicine from Newcastle University, an M.S. in the epidemiology of microbial diseases from Yale University, and a B.S. in zoology and the history of science from the University of Wisconsin–Madison. Before her time at the National Academies, Dr. Winters managed U.S. Department of State global health security programs at the Henry M. Jackson Foundation and the American Society for Microbiology, which took her to the Middle East/North Africa, South Asia, and sub-Saharan Africa.

Claire Moerder was a research associate working on the influenza consensus studies, with a focus on public health countermeasures and global coordination, partnerships, and financing. In 2015, she graduated from Virginia Tech with a B.S. in nutrition and exercise science, and has experience with special education teaching and in the sustainable jewelry industry. Since joining the National Academies, she has been working on a variety of global health topics such as violence prevention, public–private partnerships, conflict and security issues, and urban health.

Emilie Ryan-Castillo is a senior program assistant working on the new influenza consensus studies. She has a B.S. in public health from American University. She was a program assistant at FHI 360 and worked on diabetes prevention and childhood obesity research projects, helping execute several large meetings bringing together the top researchers from the U.S. Centers for Disease Control and Prevention, the U.S. National Institutes of Health, the U.S. Department of Agriculture, and the Robert Wood Johnson Foundation for the National Collaborative on Childhood Obesity Research. Recently, she was a rural community health volunteer in the Peace Corps in Benin, where she worked on improving maternal health, vaccination rates, and community outreach at a local clinic in the Borgou Department.

Patricia A. Cuff, M.S., M.P.H., is a senior program officer and directs the Global Forum on Innovation in Health Professional Education since 2012. Ms. Cuff is also working on a special COVID-related project with select academies in Africa. Ms. Cuff worked for 11 years on the African Science Academy Development Initiative, where she was the country liaison to the

Uganda National Academy of Sciences. She has directed and co-directed multiple studies at the National Academies, including *Clinical Trials During the 2014–2015 Ebola Outbreak, Options for Overseas Placement of U.S. Health Professionals,* and *Enhancing the Behavioral and Social Science Content of Medical School Curricula.* She joined the National Academies staff to work on the report *Emerging Microbial Threats to Health in the Twenty-First Century.* Earlier, Ms. Cuff worked at St. Luke's-Roosevelt Hospital Center in New York City in the field of HIV nutrition as a counselor, researcher, and lecturer on topics of adult and pediatric HIV. She received an M.S. in nutrition and an M.P.H. in population and family health from Columbia University and performed her undergraduate studies at the University of Connecticut.

Julie A. Pavlin, M.D., Ph.D., M.P.H., is the senior director of the Board on Global Health and board certified in preventive medicine and public health. She is a retired colonel in the U.S. Army with assignments including the Armed Forces Research Institute of Medical Sciences in Bangkok, Thailand, the Walter Reed Army Institute of Research, and the U.S. Army Medical Research Institute for Infectious Diseases. After she retired from active duty, she served as the deputy director of the Armed Forces Health Surveillance Center. She concentrated most of her time with the U.S. Department of Defense in the design of real-time disease surveillance systems and was a co-founder of the International Society for Disease Surveillance.

Frances Sharples served as the director of the National Academies' Board on Life Sciences until March 1, 2020, where she supervised a group of staff who developed reports, workshops, and other products dealing with the life sciences and their policy implications. Dr. Sharples joined the National Academies in October 2000. Immediately prior to that, she spent 4 years as a senior policy analyst in the Environment Division of the Office of Science and Technology Policy, Executive Office of the President. Earlier, she served in various roles in the Environmental Sciences Division of the National Laboratory in Oak Ridge, Tennessee. Dr. Sharples did her undergraduate education at Barnard College and received an M.A. and a Ph.D. from the Department of Zoology at the University of California, Davis. Dr. Sharples continues to work at the National Academies in a part-time, semi-retired mode.

Roger Yat-Nork Chung, Ph.D., M.H.S., is the inaugural National Academy of Medicine International Health Policy Fellow (2019–2021), studying the issues of health equity and social determinants of healthy longevity. He is also an appointed vice chair of the Public Health Global Challenge Steering Group of the Worldwide Universities Network, spearheading the direction of research and collaboration in public health for 23 universities. A social epidemiologist by training, Dr. Chung conceptualizes the population health and health care issues using the lens of health equity and social justice in the areas of social determinants of health, poverty and deprivation, migrants' health, patients with serious illness (including rare diseases and terminal illness), and aging-related issues of multimorbidity and long-term/end-of-life care. He has been involved in government-commissioned projects on elderly and end-of-life care, financing mechanisms for medical assistance programs, and health care resource allocation exercises. Dr. Chung obtained a B.A. in Public Health from Johns Hopkins University, an M.H.S. from the Johns Hopkins Bloomberg School of Public Health, and a Ph.D. from the School of Public Health of The University of Hong Kong. He is an assistant professor of the School of Public Health and Primary Care of the Chinese University of Hong Kong. He is also the associate director of the Institute of Health Equity and the Centre for Bioethics, a founding member of the Centre for Health Systems and Policy Research and the Research Centre for Migration and Mobility, an executive member of the Centre for Quality of Life, and an assistant professor (by courtesy) at the Institute of Ageing.

Appendix B

Committee Meeting Agendas

Committee on Global Coordination, Partnerships, and Financing Recommendations for Advancing Pandemic and Seasonal Influenza Vaccine Preparedness and Response

First Committee Meeting Agenda

March 9, 2021 (7:00–10:00 a.m. EST)
March 10, 2021 (7:00–9:00 a.m. EST)
March 11, 2021 (7:00–9:00 a.m. EST)

Meeting Objectives

- Conduct committee and staff introductions and a bias/conflict of interest discussion
- Orient the committee to the National Academies consensus study process
- Hold an open session to hear from sponsoring agency (U.S. Department of Health and Human Services' Office of Global Affairs) and the National Academy of Medicine's International Committee on Advancing Pandemic and Seasonal Influenza Preparedness and Response, on their perspective of the Statement of Task and to hear from relevant stakeholders
- Hold an open session to obtain background from speakers on the current global landscape for implementing and financing influenza vaccination and its barriers
- Discuss the Statement of Task and devise a committee work plan
- Identify information needs and future meeting topics

Tuesday, March 9, 2021

OPEN SESSION

8:25 a.m. **Welcome and Introductions**
PETER SANDS, *Committee Chair*
Executive Director
The Global Fund to Fight AIDS, Tuberculosis and Malaria

8:30 a.m. **Speaker 1 and Discussion: The International Committee on Advancing Pandemic and Seasonal Influenza Vaccine Preparedness and Response and Consensus Studies**
PRASHANT YADAV
International Committee Cochair
Senior Fellow
Center for Global Development

8:40 a.m. **Speaker 2 and Discussion: Sponsor Perspectives on the Charge to the Committee**
LARRY KERR
Director, Pandemics and Emerging Threats
Office of Global Affairs
U.S. Department of Health and Human Services

9:10 a.m. **Speaker 3 and Discussion: Envisioning Influenza at the World Health Organization: Global Frameworks and Partnerships for Influenza Vaccination**
SYLVIE BRIAND
Director, Global Infectious Hazard Preparedness
World Health Organization

9:40 a.m. **Adjourn Open Session**

Wednesday, March 10, 2021

OPEN SESSION

7:00 a.m. **Welcome and Introductions**
PETER SANDS, *Committee Chair*
Executive Director
The Global Fund to Fight AIDS, Tuberculosis and Malaria

7:05 a.m.	**Speaker 1 and Discussion: Governance and Global Collaboration for Zoonotic Influenza and Vaccines** IAN BROWN *Steering Committee Chairman* *OIE/FAO Network of Expertise on Animal Influenza (OFFLU)*
7:30 a.m.	**Speaker 2 and Discussion: Contemporary Perspectives on Pathogen Sharing: The Pandemic Influenza Preparedness (PIP) Framework and the Nagoya Protocol** SANGEETA SHASHIKANT *Legal Advisor* *Third World Network*
8:00 a.m.	**Speaker 3 and Discussion: Global Partnerships for Influenza Vaccination** JEREMY FARRAR *Director* *Wellcome Trust*
8:30 a.m.	**Speaker 4 and Discussion: The Global Supply of Influenza Vaccines: Governance, Progress, and Areas for Growth** MARIE-PAULE KIENY *Director of Research* *Institut National de la Santé et la Recherche Médicale (INSERM)*
8:55 a.m.	**Closing Remarks and Adjourn Day 2** PETER SANDS, *Committee Chair* *Executive Director* *The Global Fund to Fight AIDS, Tuberculosis and Malaria*

Second Committee Meeting Agenda

April 9, 2021 (8:00–11:00 a.m. EDT)
April 16, 2021 (7:00–10:00 a.m. EDT)

Friday, April 9, 2021

OPEN SESSION

8:55 a.m.	**Welcome and Introductions**
9:00 a.m.	**Speaker 1 and Discussion: Update on Global Manufacturing Capacity and Access Barriers for Influenza Vaccines** THOMAS CUENI *Chief Executive Officer, International Federation of Pharmaceutical Manufacturers & Associations (IFPMA)*
9:35 a.m.	**Speaker 2 and Discussion: Potential Financing and Coordination Mechanisms for Pandemic Vaccination** NICOLE LURIE *Strategic Advisor to the Chief Executive Officer, Coalition for Epidemic Preparedness Innovations (CEPI)*
10:10 a.m.	**Closing Remarks**

Friday, April 16, 2021

OPEN SESSION

7:00 a.m.	**Welcome and Introductions**
7:05 a.m.	**Speaker 1: Governance Structures and Barriers in the African Region for Influenza Vaccine Manufacturing** PATRICK TIPPOO *Executive Committee Vice President, Developing Country Vaccine Manufacturing Network (DCVMN)* *Founding Member, African Vaccine Manufacturers Initiative (AVMI)* *Head of Science and Innovation, Biovac*
7:35 a.m.	**Speaker 2: Current Challenges and Coordination Mechanisms in the MENA Region for Influenza Surveillance and Access** SALAH AL AWAIDY *Communicable Diseases Advisor,* *Ministry of Health, Oman*
8:00 a.m.	**Speaker 3: The Developing Country Vaccine Manufacturers Network (DCVMN) and Current Challenges in Brazil for Influenza Vaccine Manufacturing** TIAGO ROCCA *Strategic Partnerships and Business Development Manager,* *Instituto Butantan* *Executive Committee Member, DCVMN*
8:30 a.m.	**Closing Remarks**

Third Committee Meeting Agenda

May 6, 2021 (8:00–10:00 a.m. EDT): *Three simultaneous working group sessions*
May 7, 2021 (9:00–11:00 a.m. EDT): *Three simultaneous working group sessions*
May 11, 2021 (1:00–1:45 p.m. EDT): *Single working group session*
May 14, 2021 (8:00–11:00 a.m. EDT): *Full committee session*

Meeting Objectives

- Hold open sessions to obtain background from speakers on the current barriers for effective global health governance for pandemic influenza vaccination, with a focus on pathogen sharing regulations, technology transfer partnerships, and global access and financing
- Hold working group deliberations to form initial recommendations
- Hold whole-committee meeting to discuss initial recommendations and next steps

Thursday, May 6, 2021

OPEN SESSION 1: TECHNOLOGY AND MANUFACTURING WORKING GROUP

8:25 a.m. **Welcome and Introductions**
BRUCE GELLIN
Director, Global Immunization
Sabin Vaccine Institute

8:30 a.m. **Speaker 1: Public–Private Partnerships for Influenza Vaccine Development and Manufacturing and the Center for Infectious Disease Research and Policy's (CIDRAP's) Influenza Vaccine Research and Development Road Map**
JOSEPH BRESEE
Associate Director, Global Health Affairs, Influenza Division
Director, Partnership for Influenza Vaccine Introduction
U.S. Centers for Disease Control and Prevention
Director, Global Funders Consortium for Universal Influenza Vaccine Development

8:55 a.m. **Closing Remarks**

Friday, May 7, 2021

OPEN SESSION: PATHOGEN SHARING WORKING GROUP

9:30 a.m. **Welcome and Introductions**
ALEXANDRA PHELAN
Assistant Professor
Center for Global Health Science and Security
Georgetown University

9:35 a.m. **Speaker 1: Speed and Equity for Pathogen and Vaccine Sharing at the World Health Organization**
STEVEN SOLOMON
Principal Legal Officer,
World Health Organization

10:00 a.m. **Speaker 2: Environmental Health Law, the Nagoya Protocol, and Influenza Pathogen Sharing**
JORGE E. VIÑUALES
Harold Samuel Chair of Law and Environmental Policy
Founder and Former Director, Cambridge Centre for Environment, Energy and Natural Resource Government,
Cambridge University

10:25 a.m. **Closing Remarks**

Friday, May 7, 2021

OPEN SESSION 2: TECHNOLOGY AND MANUFACTURING WORKING GROUP

9:00 a.m. **Welcome and Introductions**
BRUCE GELLIN
Director, Global Immunization
Sabin Vaccine Institute

9:05 a.m. **Speaker 1: The Coalition for Epidemic Preparedness and Innovations' (CEPI's) Role as a Broker and Facilitator of Manufacturing Partnerships**
James Robinson
CEPI Scientific Advisory Committee Vice Chair
James Robinson Biologics Consulting

9:30 a.m. **Closing Remarks**

Friday, May 7, 2021

OPEN SESSION: VACCINE ACCESS AND FINANCING WORKING GROUP

9:00 a.m. Opening Remarks
Amanda Glassman
Senior Fellow and Executive Vice President
Center for Global Engagement

9:05 a.m. **Speaker 1: Lessons from Economic Theory: Developing Quick Pandemic Vaccines and Distributing Them Equitably**
Gavin Yamey
Associate Director for Policy and Professor of the Practice of Global Health and Public Policy
Director, Center for Policy Impact in Global Health
Duke Global Health Institute

David McAdams
Professor of Business Administration, Fuqua School of Business
Professor of Economics, Economics Department
Duke University

Osondu Ogbuoji
Assistant Research Professor
Deputy Director, Center for Policy Impact in Global Health
Duke Global Health Institute

9:30 a.m.	**Speaker 2: The World Bank's Post-Pandemic Emergency Financing Facility Agenda for Financing Pandemic Preparedness and Economic Theory for Incentivizing Vaccine Access** MUHAMMAD ALI PATE *Global Director,* *Health, Nutrition and Population (HNP) Global Practice* *World Bank*
10:00 a.m.	**Speaker 3: Europe's Experiences with Procuring COVID-19 Vaccines** ANDRZEJ RYS *Director for Health Systems, Medical Products and Innovation* *Directorate-General for Health and Food Safety, European Commission*
10:20 a.m.	**Closing Remarks**

Tuesday, May 11, 2021

OPEN SESSION 3: TECHNOLOGY AND MANUFACTURING WORKING GROUP

9:00 a.m.	**Welcome and Introductions** BRUCE GELLIN *Director, Global Immunization* *Sabin Vaccine Institute*
1:00 p.m.	**Speaker 1: Lessons Learned from the Global Action Plan for Influenza Vaccines' (GAP's) Technology Transfer Partnerships and the Biomedical Advanced Research and Development Authority's (BARDA's) International Influenza Vaccine Technology Manufacturing Capacity Program** JULIE SCHAFER *Chief Technology Officer* *Flu Lab* ERIN SPARROW *Technical Officer* *World Health Organization*
1:45 p.m.	**Closing Remarks**